How to
Get a Job
in Health Care

How to
Get a Job
in Health Care

ROBERT H. ZEDLITZ

THOMSON

DELMAR LEARNING

Australia   Canada   Mexico   Singapore   Spain   United   Kingdom   United States

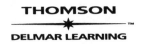

How to Get a Job in Health Care
by Robert H. Zedlitz

Executive Director Health Care Business Unit:
William Brottmiller

Executive Editor:
Cathy L. Esperti

Acquisitions Editor:
Sherry Gomoll

Technology Project Manager:
Joseph Saba/Victoria Moore

Executive Marketing Manager:
Dawn F. Gerrain

Editorial Assistant:
Jennifer Conklin

Production Editor:
James Zayicek

For permission to use material from this text or product,
contact us by
Tel   (800) 730-2214
Fax   (800) 730-2215
www.thomsonrights.com

Library of Congress Cataloging-in-Publication Data

Zedlitz, Robert H.
    How to get a job in health care / Robert H. Zedlitz.
        p. cm.
    ISBN-10: 0-7668-4193-6
    ISBN-13: 978-0-7668-4193-2
    1. Allied health personnel--Vocational guidance. I. Title.
R697.A4Z43 2002
610.69'53--dc21   2002022297

NOTICE TO THE READER

CONTENTS

PREFACE

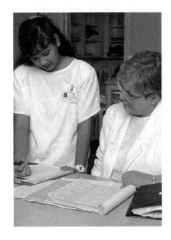

Health care is one of the largest and fastest growing industries in the United States. By the year 2008 health services employment is projected to increase to 13,600,000 with over 2,800,000 new jobs. The need for increased health care is in part the result of advanced medical technology and changes in public attitude about health care. Great advances have been made in medical knowledge. Americans today appreciate the benefits provided by prevention of health problems. This attitude has helped develop a broad area of new services, health maintenance organizations, and employment opportunities. Modern medicine and health care awareness have enabled more people to live longer. The elderly make up a larger percentage of the population than ever before. Our aging population will create many changes and open up new areas of the health care industry. Older people usually need more, and different kinds of, health care services than younger people.

Projections indicate that the number of jobs related to health care will increase substantially within the next decade. It is projected that health care services will account for almost one-fifth of all job growth through the year 2005. This presents a tremendous employment opportunity for trained men and women of every age and background. *How to Get a Job in Health Care* is designed to help you get your first job—or move to another health care job. *How to Get a Job in Health Care* also tells you how to leave your job gracefully with excellent references, should a better career opportunity present itself.

The health care industry offers many jobs that are challenging. Examples include the positions held by physicians, nurses, medical and dental assistants, technicians, technologists, or therapists. In addition, many health care workers are employed as support personnel performing clerical or maintenance tasks, or as workers in closely related industries. Different jobs are being created as the nature and scope of health care change and evolve. Remember, you are not locked into any one particular job in the health care industry. It will be possible for you to make a job change with further training and education. You will certainly discover that a career in the health care industry affords you responsibility—and rewards you with advancement.

Whether you are getting your first job or contemplating an employment change, there are many interesting positions in the health care industry that can lead to a rewarding career. Among them are

dental assistant

dental hygienist

dental lab technician

dental secretary

dietitian

electrocardiograph technician

home health aide

medical lab assistant

medical receptionist

medical record technician

medical transcriptionist

nurse (RN)

nursing assistant

orthopedic therapy assistant

paramedic

pediatric assistant

physical therapy assistant

psychiatric assistant

surgical technician

vision care technician

X-ray technician

How to Get a Job in Health Care provides an easy-to-follow, step-by-step guide for obtaining a career position in the health care industry. It offers you an employment process, materials, and techniques to obtain the job you want. In addition, it offers a graceful method to use when changing a health care position.

STUDENT'S MATERIALS

How to Get a Job in Health Care consists of an employment manual divided into four sections. Sections 1 and 2 cover how to get and leave a job, while Section 3 activities provide documents necessary for success in the health care job process. Section 4 contains keys to using the accompanying CD-ROM. Your personal guide, *How to Get a Job in Health Care* is vital to success in gaining employment. You will have the advantage of being prepared because you will have acquired the student's employment manual and copies of important employment documents, saved in an employment portfolio and as files to a computer disk.

Section 1: Getting a Job in Health Care

Section 1 of the manual, which contains seven steps with activities, forms an effective, workable guide for actually landing the position, as well as references you want in the health care industry. Because the material is divided into self-explanatory parts, precious preparation time is saved. Individualized material allows you to progress at your own pace. At the beginning of each step in Section 1, a summary of its important features provides a quick review and guide to the contents.

Section 2: Leaving a Health Care Job...Gracefully

Section 2 of *How to Get a Job in Health Care* contains valuable advice and insight concerning how to leave a health care job gracefully with excellent references. There is far more to leaving a job than saying, "I quit." This section includes procedures and activities that will end your job on a positive note.

Section 3: Getting and Leaving a Job in Health Care—Activities

Section 3 of this manual contains self-directed activities to complete each step of Section 1 and Section 2. The instructions in Sections 1 and 2 are reinforced by 15 appropriate, meaningful activities that allow you to participate while being led systematically through the text. The activities make *How to Get a Job in Health Care* action-orientated.

The activities are:

Activity 1 Checklist of Employment Power Words and Phrases
Activity 2 Writing Health Care Job Objectives
Activity 3 Constructing a Health Care Resume
Activity 4 Constructing a Health Care Reference List
Activity 5 Writing a Health Care Cover Letter
Activity 6 Completing a Health Care Employment Application
Activity 7 Finding Health Care Job Leads
Activity 8 Researching a Health Care Facility
Activity 9 Answering Interview Questions
Activity 10 Health Care Case Study Questions
Activity 11 Preparing a Health Care Post Interview Letter
Activity 12 Health Care Case Study—Decision Time
Activity 13 Writing a Health Care Resignation Letter
Activity 14 Health Care Exit Conversation
Activity 15 Constructing a Health Care Reference Letter

Employment Portfolio

As each activity in Section 3 of *How to Get a Job in Health Care* is completed, a copy can be placed in an employment portfolio. The employment portfolio can be any type of your choosing. It can be as simple as a file folder, which establishes a record of valuable papers necessary for employment in the health care industry. Your employment portfolio, with the completed activities, will provide guidelines for securing and leaving health care jobs now and in your future health care career. An employment portfolio containing all of these materials will be extremely convenient in the future, providing an easy and convenient access to useful employment aids.

Keying Featured Documents

Throughout *How to Get a Job in Health Care* you are encouraged to key featured documents using word processing software and saving all of your document files on the same computer disk. Your computer disk will allow instant use and easy up-date. Featured documents include your

- resume
- reference list
- cover letter
- post interview letter
- resignation letter
- reference letter

Section 4: CD-ROM

Your accompanying CD-ROM contains 18 files you may use to supplement your *How to Get a Job in Health Care* activities and create your resume and letter documents. After you complete selected activity practice sheets in Section 3, you may use your personal CD-ROM to create these documents. The CD-ROM icon shown with activities directs you to Section 4 for using the CD-ROM files.

Your CD-ROM also includes the Health Care Resume Generator. After entering your personal information, this easy-to-use software will generate a variety of personalized resumes and cover letters designed specifically to help you find a rewarding job in the health care field.

A Tool for Your Success

The health care industry is rewarding. The number of new jobs and services is rapidly increasing. Few industries offer such diverse employment opportunities. Many geographic areas, such as densely populated, inner-city areas and thinly populated, rural areas, are experiencing a shortage of health care workers. Due to the shortage of health care workers, and the need for employers to attract qualified health care workers, benefit programs are being improved. Opportunities such as tuition reimbursement, flex-time, and job-sharing are offered. To find the most rewarding job in health care, consider the many influences and changes in the field. Completing *How to Get a Job in Health Care* will add to your confidence in this challenge. This manual makes employment in the health care industry a reality, and leaving your job a positive career move.

Note to the Instructor

In addition to the students' materials, an *Instructor's Manual* with valuable health care information is available to you, the educator. The *Instructor's Manual to Accompany How to Get a Job in Health Care* contains detailed strategies that help students complete the activities provided in this manual. There are helpful suggestions for teaching each part of the student's manual. Other strategies ensure that the student is thoroughly prepared for the health care industry employment process. These points include how to effectively

- present a resume to a prospective health care employer
- write job objectives
- read an employment advertisement
- understand various health care employment applications

- give positive or neutral reasons for leaving a job
- answer the salary questions
- use a health care business annual report
- relate one's own experience to a specific health care opening during an interview.

The *Instructor's Manual* also contains transparency masters that the instructor may display for classroom use, and two that are appropriate as handouts for student activities. There are activity transparency masters that serve as formatting guides for the resume, reference list, cover letter, post-interview letter, reference letter, and resignation letter. These important aids will help the student key perfect health care industry documents. Several other transparency masters offer useful information for class work or future health care industry employment.

About the Author

With over 40 years of instructional experience in business, work, and career education, Robert H. Zedlitz understands what is required for students to gain employment. At present, the author is involved in Career and Work Experience Education in Fremont, California.

In addition, he is a past member of the Work Experience Education Consortium Committee for the California State Department of Education.

ACKNOWLEDGMENTS

A special thank you to all the reviewers who offer many wonderful suggestions.

Amelia Broussard, PhD, RN, MPH
Associate Professor of Health Care Management
Clayton College & State University
Jasper, GA

Patti Biro, BS, MEd
Director, Health Care Programs
Del Mar College
Corpus Cristi, TX

Celeste Fenton, BA, MEd, ABD-PhD
Manager, Career Planning and Placement
Hillsborough Community College
Tampa, FL

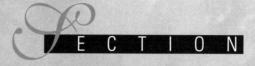

SECTION

1

Getting a Job
in Health Care

INTRODUCTION

Almost everyone needs to polish basic job-hunting skills. This employment guide, *How to Get a Job in Health Care,* offers students, the recent graduate, or person who plans to enter or return to the workforce an easy-to-follow, step-by-step guide for obtaining a career position in the health care industry.

The seven steps in Section 1, Getting a Job in Health Care, follow, along with a summary of what each step includes.

Step 1: Health Care Resume

This step deals with important information about preparing resumes. Four sample resumes and a reference list are included to ensure that the job candidate's resumes are effective.

Step 2: Health Care Cover Letter

This step deals with cover letters and their importance in looking for a health care job. Sample cover letters and instructions tell what a cover letter should say and how to write one.

Step 3: Health Care Employment Application

This step deals with what health care employers look for in employment applications. A sample employment application and two practice application forms are included.

Step 4: Finding and Researching a Health Care Job and Facility

This step outlines the most important sources of health care job leads and how to pursue them. It also teaches the job candidate how to research a health care facility and a job title.

Step 5: How to Prepare for a Health Care Interview

This step tells what to take to a health care job interview and how to appear your best. Included are 12 of the most common interview questions and suggested answers.

Step 6: During the Health Care Interview

This step tells what to do during an interview. An interview case study, activity, questions, and a "Do's and Don'ts" checklist are included.

Step 7: After the Health Care Interview

This step outlines what to do after a health care interview to give the job candidate an edge over competitors. Three types of contacts are explored, including a successful post-interview letter.

STEP 1
HEALTH CARE RESUME (PERSONAL DATASHEET)

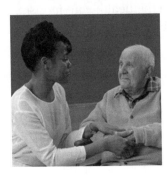

In this step you will find

- the definition of resume (pronounced REH-zoo-may).
- reasons why your health care resume is important.
- instructions for writing your health care resume.
- an activity checklist of employment power words and phrases.
- four sample health care resumes and writing activities.
- an activity to construct a health care reference list.

WHAT IS A RESUME?

A resume is a personal data sheet. It is a short summary of important facts about you. These facts help a health care employer decide whether or not you are an appropriate candidate for medical-related jobs. Resumes are usually sent to potential employers with a cover letter asking for an interview.

Any person who is serious about seeking a job in the health care field should always have a well-thought-out, up-to-date, and well-prepared resume. Remember, the resume creates a first impression and may get you the health care interview. It must be accurate and error free.

WHY IS YOUR HEALTH CARE RESUME IMPORTANT?

You should prepare a health care resume for the following reasons.

- **To help you complete a health care employment application quickly and accurately.** An employment application is a form used by many medical organizations to gather information about a job candidate.

- **To demonstrate your potential as a health care worker.** Resumes provide additional information and reflect a health care job applicant's qualifications better than an employment application. Always give a health care employer a copy of your resume along with your completed employment application if you do not have an interview planned when you submit the application. Often this extra fact sheet can help you get an interview at a later date.

- **To show a health care employer you are organized, prepared, and serious about getting a job.** Health care employers often consider you an above-average candidate for a job because you included a resume.

- **To feel self-assured during an interview because important facts and dates are in front of you.** Having a resume helps you feel professional and adds to your self-confidence.

- **To mail or fax to potential health care employers with whom you would like to arrange an interview.** You can mail or fax copies of your resume to more health care employers than you can visit. This saves you time and money. Remember, the primary purpose of a health care resume is to convince someone to interview you for a health care job.

- **To distribute to relatives, friends, guidance counselors, teachers, character references, and other persons who are willing to help you find a health care job.** Your resume gives these important people a clear picture of your qualifications. It also acts as a constant reminder that you are seeking health care employment. A health care job lead could very well result from one of these close contacts.

WHAT SHOULD BE INCLUDED ON A RESUME?

Resumes are written in many different styles. Four resume styles are included here: standard, chronological, functional, and combination. However, there are basic elements that must be included in any resume style. These basic elements include personal information, education, work experience, qualifications for the job position, and references. Carefully read the A–H description sections of Figure 1-1-1. See how each description section compares to the same A–H sections of the standard style resume, Figure 1-1-2.

Now examine the remaining three resume styles. Figure 1-1-3 is a chronological resume, Figure 1-1-4 is a functional resume, and Figure 1-1-5 is a combination resume. Notice they are written in different styles, but all contain the same basic elements of successful resumes.

WHAT RESUME STYLE IS BEST FOR YOU?

Good judgment is necessary to determine what to include in your health care resume. Study the description of the four resume samples and decide which style best describes your work experience and skills.

- **Standard resume:** Look at Figure 1-1-2, the sample standard resume. Notice the standard resume information is organized by category. This makes the standard resume easy to develop. You can quickly fill in the blanks under each heading. It clearly shows a prospective health care employer your personal information, job objective, work experience, education, and work skills. A standard resume can also emphasize memberships, honors, and special skills. A first-time employee, and/or recent graduate, might feel more comfortable developing this type of resume.

- **Chronological resume:** Look at Figure 1-1-3, the sample chronological resume. Notice the chronological resume lists experiences in order of time. Your work and educational experience are dated with the most recent experience given first. Use this style to show steady employment without gaps or a great number of job changes. At the top of your chronological resume place your job objective, followed by a description of your job objective qualifications.

- **Functional resume:** Look at Figure 1-1-4, the sample functional resume. Notice that the functional resume is a series of paragraphs that identify a job candidate's most important work skills. You can arrange your resume paragraphs in order of importance to your job objective. List your most important work-related experience first. Use this format when you have gaps in employment and lack experience directly related to your job objective.

● **Combination resume:** Look at Figure 1-1-5, the sample combination resume. Notice the combination resume combines chronological and functional resume styles. It gives the work experience directly related to the job opening by most recent date first and arranges the resume information in paragraphs. Specific job skills are listed to capture the employers' attention for a match with the position requirements. Use this format if you have limited experience or want to highlight your accomplishments directed to a particular job opening.

Creating Your Perfect Health Care Resume

To create a professional looking health care resume, study the sample resumes. Notice the margin and spacing guidelines. See the following box for an explanation of the formatting guidelines on each resume. Keep your resume readable and organized by section headings and add space between sections. Keep in mind, though, you want to limit your resume to one or two pages.

FORMATTING GUIDELINES

Spacing: Correct spacing between parts of a document is indicated as:

2S (Double space): Insert one blank line and type on the second line. Press the return bar twice to double space between sections.

4S (Quadruple space): Type on every fourth line with three blank lines between each line. Press the return bar four times to quadruple space between sections.

Margins: Correct top, side, and bottom margins are stated in inches from the edge of the document to the point where keying should begin or end. Top margins are also indicated with the proper line to begin keying on.

Call-outs and Notes: Explanatory information is linked to sections of documents with an arrow or with letter markers like this one: Look for the note that accompanies a document for an explanation of each marker.

Guidelines for Creating A
Standard Health Care Resume

Ⓐ PERSONAL INFORMATION

List your name, address, telephone and fax number, and E-mail address. The prospective health care employer may need to know some additional facts about you, but this information must stay within the bounds of your state's fair employment laws. The prospective employer will use this information to contact you.

Ⓑ JOB OBJECTIVE

The job objective states the health care position you are seeking. It should be a clearly and concisely written sentence of your job goal. For example: "To work as a licensed Vocational Nurse at a well-managed convalescent hospital." A well-written job objective can also include a career goal or the ultimate job position you would like to achieve in the health care field. Your job objective and career goal should be closely related. For example: "To work for a large hospital as a Medical Record Technician, which could lead to a position as a Medical Record Supervisor."

Ⓒ EDUCATION

List the schools you have attended in reverse chronological order (most recent first). Include dates of attendance, the name and location of the schools, the curriculum studied (general education, medical assisting, dental assisting, college preparatory, etc.), and the degree or diploma earned. Also list any courses that relate to your career objective. High school records may or may not be listed. If you are still attending school, place your expected graduation month and year in parenthesis next to your diploma or degree. For example: Licensed Vocational Nurse Certificate (June, 20—).

Ⓓ WORK EXPERIENCE

List all full-time, part-time, summer, or volunteer jobs. Be sure to list any internship. Present your work experience in reverse chronological order (most recent first). Include dates of employment, names and locations of the health care facilities or organizations, names of your supervisor, job titles, work responsibilities, and duties. Show how your previous work and skills apply to your job objective and career goal.

Ⓔ MEMBERSHIPS

Include memberships in professional health care organizations or other career-related clubs and associations. This shows that you are willing to donate valuable time to worthy causes without compensation. Use good judgment, however, before listing religious, political, or any other sensitive organization memberships. You are not required to disclose any memberships that are not job related. If you have no memberships, eliminate this section.

Ⓕ HONORS

List any honors, special certificates of achievement, and awards you have received. If you had a high class ranking, record it here. If you have no honors or special awards, eliminate this section.

Ⓖ SPECIAL SKILLS

List any special skills that you wish to highlight even if they are not job related. A prospective employer should be aware of all your talents. For example: reading, writing, and speaking knowledge of Spanish. If you have no special skills, eliminate this section.

Ⓗ REFERENCES

Place the following statement at the bottom of your resume: "References available on request." Key and provide a separate list of references when you interview. The name, business title (if any), company or organization, address, and telephone number of your references are usually required. Be sure to ask permission of those references you plan to provide. Include former employers, instructors, doctors, nurses, or friends well established in business or the health care field who know your character and accomplishments. See Figure 1-1-6 for an example of a reference list.

Figure 1-1-1 Standard Resume Descriptions for Figure 1-1-2

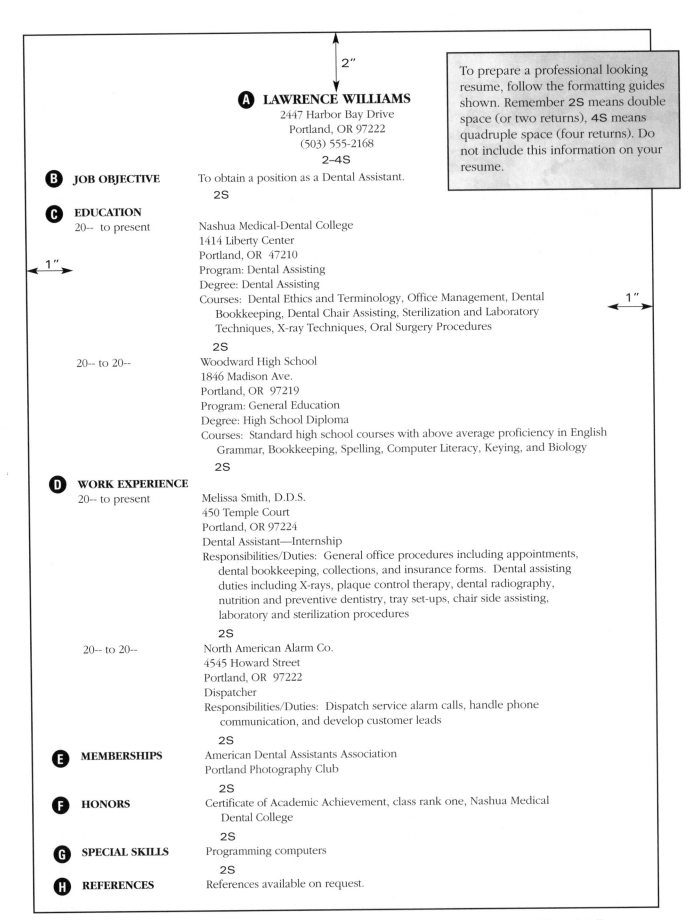

2"

A **LAWRENCE WILLIAMS**
2447 Harbor Bay Drive
Portland, OR 97222
(503) 555-2168
2–4S

To prepare a professional looking resume, follow the formatting guides shown. Remember **2S** means double space (or two returns), **4S** means quadruple space (four returns). Do not include this information on your resume.

B **JOB OBJECTIVE**   To obtain a position as a Dental Assistant.
2S

C **EDUCATION**
20-- to present
Nashua Medical-Dental College
1414 Liberty Center
Portland, OR 47210
Program: Dental Assisting
Degree: Dental Assisting
Courses: Dental Ethics and Terminology, Office Management, Dental Bookkeeping, Dental Chair Assisting, Sterilization and Laboratory Techniques, X-ray Techniques, Oral Surgery Procedures
2S

1"

1"

20-- to 20--
Woodward High School
1846 Madison Ave.
Portland, OR 97219
Program: General Education
Degree: High School Diploma
Courses: Standard high school courses with above average proficiency in English Grammar, Bookkeeping, Spelling, Computer Literacy, Keying, and Biology
2S

D **WORK EXPERIENCE**
20-- to present
Melissa Smith, D.D.S.
450 Temple Court
Portland, OR 97224
Dental Assistant—Internship
Responsibilities/Duties: General office procedures including appointments, dental bookkeeping, collections, and insurance forms. Dental assisting duties including X-rays, plaque control therapy, dental radiography, nutrition and preventive dentistry, tray set-ups, chair side assisting, laboratory and sterilization procedures
2S

20-- to 20--
North American Alarm Co.
4545 Howard Street
Portland, OR 97222
Dispatcher
Responsibilities/Duties: Dispatch service alarm calls, handle phone communication, and develop customer leads
2S

E **MEMBERSHIPS**   American Dental Assistants Association
Portland Photography Club
2S

F **HONORS**   Certificate of Academic Achievement, class rank one, Nashua Medical Dental College
2S

G **SPECIAL SKILLS**   Programming computers
2S

H **REFERENCES**   References available on request.

Figure 1-1-2 Sample Standard Resume. Note: Circled letters coincide with guideline explanations on previous page.

2″

JOAN DE CAMPO
5151 Center Street
Springfield, Illinois 48264
(217) 555-3238
2–4S

JOB OBJECTIVE

2S

To join a leading health clinic as a Medical Record Technician. Future goal
is to manage a multidoctor medical facility.

2S

QUALIFICATIONS

2S

Clinical Experience: Patient intake; numbering, filing and preservation
of medical records; collecting medical care and census data for statistical
purposes; computing and preparing statistical reports; transcribing medical
reports; coding of diseases and operations by standard classifications; recording
and reporting vital statistics; assisting with quality insurance programs;
assisting administrative and medical staff

2S

Proficient in oral and written English, oral Spanish, mathematics, keying
(80 WPM) and word processing skills

2S

Graduated in upper five percent of my class, June, 20--, Chicago Community
College, Chicago, IL. Received an A. A. Degree in Medical Record Technology.
Eligible for the American Medical Record Association examination for designation
as an Accredited Record Technician (ART), September 15, 20--. Student member
of the American Medical Record Association.

2S

Graduated June, 20-- from Mission High School, Springfield, IL, with
a science major.

2S

EMPLOYERS

2S

May, 20-- to present	Marine Midland Trust Company
	Springfield, IL
	Merchant Teller
	2S
May to June, 20--	Allen Memorial Hospital
	Springfield, IL
	Directed Internship
	2S
February to April, 20--	St. Mary's HMO
	Springfield, IL
	Directed Internship
	2S
April, 20-- to March, 20--	Philan Photo Finishing
	Springfield, IL
	Salesperson

2S

REFERENCES

2S

References available on request.

1″   1″

Figure 1-1-3 Sample Chronological Resume

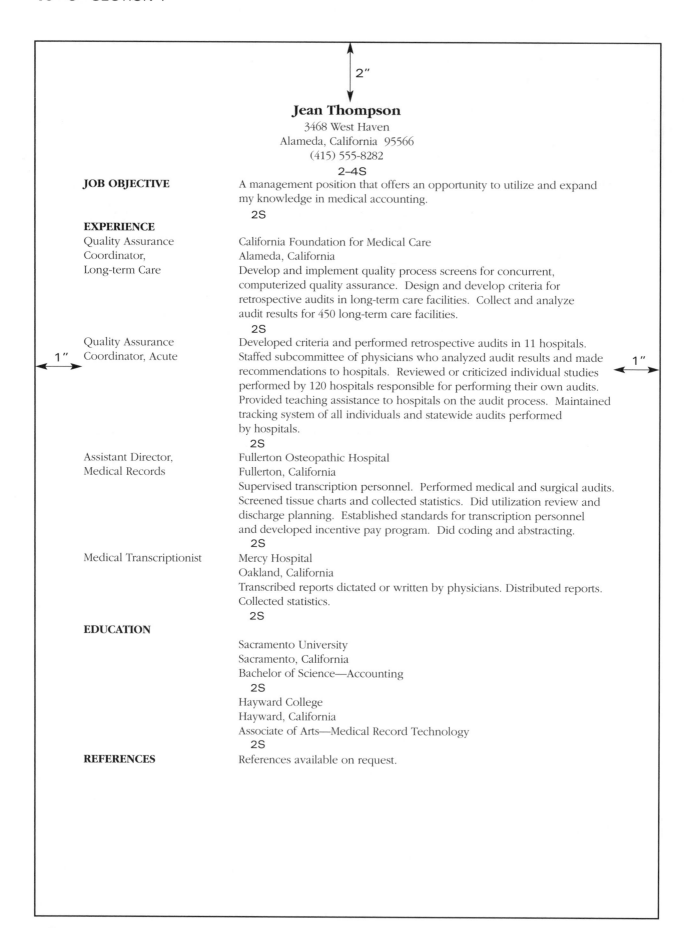

2″

Jean Thompson
3468 West Haven
Alameda, California 95566
(415) 555-8282
2–4S

JOB OBJECTIVE   A management position that offers an opportunity to utilize and expand my knowledge in medical accounting.
2S

EXPERIENCE

Quality Assurance Coordinator, Long-term Care
California Foundation for Medical Care
Alameda, California
Develop and implement quality process screens for concurrent, computerized quality assurance. Design and develop criteria for retrospective audits in long-term care facilities. Collect and analyze audit results for 450 long-term care facilities.
2S

1″

Quality Assurance Coordinator, Acute
Developed criteria and performed retrospective audits in 11 hospitals. Staffed subcommittee of physicians who analyzed audit results and made recommendations to hospitals. Reviewed or criticized individual studies performed by 120 hospitals responsible for performing their own audits. Provided teaching assistance to hospitals on the audit process. Maintained tracking system of all individuals and statewide audits performed by hospitals.

1″

2S

Assistant Director, Medical Records
Fullerton Osteopathic Hospital
Fullerton, California
Supervised transcription personnel. Performed medical and surgical audits. Screened tissue charts and collected statistics. Did utilization review and discharge planning. Established standards for transcription personnel and developed incentive pay program. Did coding and abstracting.
2S

Medical Transcriptionist
Mercy Hospital
Oakland, California
Transcribed reports dictated or written by physicians. Distributed reports. Collected statistics.
2S

EDUCATION

Sacramento University
Sacramento, California
Bachelor of Science—Accounting
2S
Hayward College
Hayward, California
Associate of Arts—Medical Record Technology
2S

REFERENCES   References available on request.

Figure 1-1-4 Sample Functional Resume

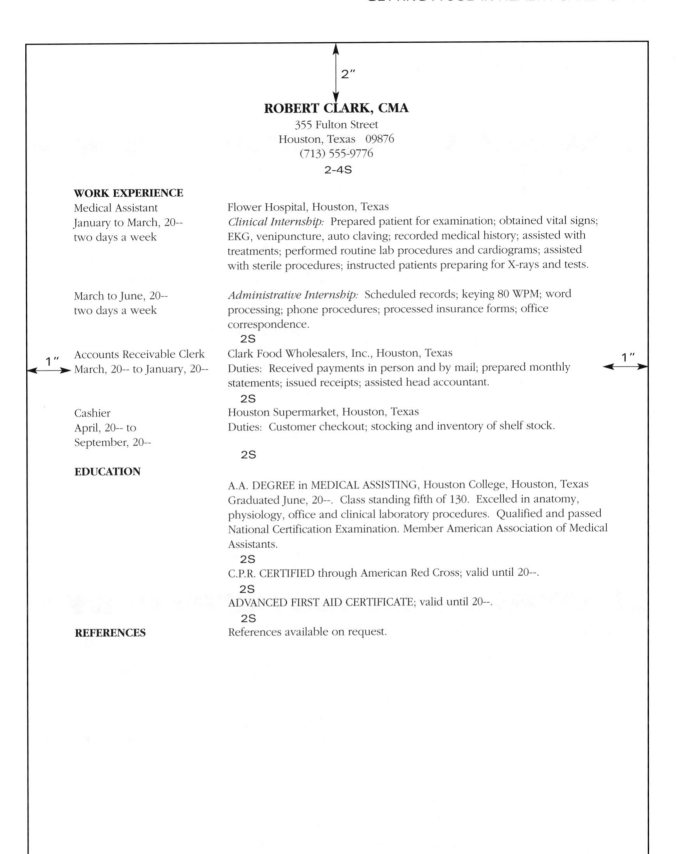

2"

ROBERT CLARK, CMA
355 Fulton Street
Houston, Texas   09876
(713) 555-9776
2-4S

1"

1"

WORK EXPERIENCE

Medical Assistant
January to March, 20--
two days a week

Flower Hospital, Houston, Texas
Clinical Internship: Prepared patient for examination; obtained vital signs; EKG, venipuncture, auto claving; recorded medical history; assisted with treatments; performed routine lab procedures and cardiograms; assisted with sterile procedures; instructed patients preparing for X-rays and tests.

March to June, 20--
two days a week

Administrative Internship: Scheduled records; keying 80 WPM; word processing; phone procedures; processed insurance forms; office correspondence.
2S

Accounts Receivable Clerk
March, 20-- to January, 20--

Clark Food Wholesalers, Inc., Houston, Texas
Duties: Received payments in person and by mail; prepared monthly statements; issued receipts; assisted head accountant.
2S

Cashier
April, 20-- to
September, 20--

Houston Supermarket, Houston, Texas
Duties: Customer checkout; stocking and inventory of shelf stock.

2S

EDUCATION

A.A. DEGREE in MEDICAL ASSISTING, Houston College, Houston, Texas Graduated June, 20--. Class standing fifth of 130. Excelled in anatomy, physiology, office and clinical laboratory procedures. Qualified and passed National Certification Examination. Member American Association of Medical Assistants.
2S
C.P.R. CERTIFIED through American Red Cross; valid until 20--.
2S
ADVANCED FIRST AID CERTIFICATE; valid until 20--.
2S

REFERENCES

References available on request.

Figure 1-1-5 Sample Combination Resume

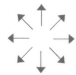

Activity Time!
Refer to Section 3—Activities.

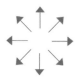

ACTIVITY 1

CHECKLIST OF EMPLOYMENT POWER WORDS AND PHRASES

Remove Activity 1, Checklist of Health Care Employment Power Words and Phrases, found in Section 3. This important checklist can be used to complete Steps 1–7 in Section 1 and Steps 1–3 in Section 2 of this manual. Carefully read the directions and complete this activity. When you have completed this activity to your satisfaction show it to your instructor for evaluation. Now start your employment portfolio. Place in it your completed activity. These are assertive words and phrases that can help you write an effective health care resume, cover letter, employment application, post-interview letter, and reference letter. These completed documents also will be kept in your employment portfolio for you to keep for future reference in your employment process.

Activity Time!
Refer to Section 3—Activities.

ACTIVITY 2

WRITING HEALTH CARE JOB OBJECTIVES

Notice that three of the sample resumes contain a job objective. A job objective may identify a specific health care job title, a type of medical-related work, or a health care career goal. If you know of a specific health care job opening, include a job objective specific to that opening in your resume. You should structure the content of your resume to the particular job opening as well.

Following are examples of health care job objectives.
- To obtain a laboratory assistant position.
- To work as an EKG technician for a hospital.
- To be hired in an entry-level position as a hospital unit coordinator.
- To join a private practice as an office medical assistant.

Notice these job objectives are clearly and concisely written. Now, remove the Activity 2 worksheet in Section 3. This worksheet includes three help-wanted advertisements. After each ad, write a job objective that would be appropriate for the health care job described. Then write a job objective for yourself for the health care job you want. After you have completed the job objectives worksheet to your satisfaction, show it to your instructor for evaluation. Place it in your employment portfolio for future reference.

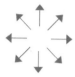

Activity Time!

Refer to Section 3—Activities.

CD-ROM

See Section 4 for directions.

ACTIVITY 3

CONSTRUCTING A HEALTH CARE RESUME

You are now ready to construct your resume. See Figure 1-1-2 through Figure 1-1-5. Observe the different styles in which the resume samples are written: standard, chronological, functional, and combination. Carefully examine each of these resumes and select a resume style that matches your work experience and skills. Remove the Activity 3 worksheet in Section 3 that correlates to the resume style you have selected. Fill in the spaces. This activity will require time and research to present as good an image of yourself as possible. It is important that you put forth your best effort in this activity. Health care employers will judge you on how thoroughly the facts are presented. However, do limit your resume to one or two pages. You are encouraged to use your own creative skills when developing a resume. You may wish to design your own resume format using a combination of the various styles presented in this step.

After you have completed the resume worksheet to your satisfaction, show it to your instructor for evaluation. Then follow the formatting guidelines in this step to complete your final resume. After you key a final resume, print several copies in the style you have selected. Use a good grade of white 8 1/2" x 11" bond paper to print your final resume. Photocopies are acceptable if they are clearly reproduced. Professional copies can be ordered from a copy center. Look in the Yellow Pages under "Printers" or "Printing." Place your final printed resumes and the computer disk on which you saved your resume file in your employment portfolio.

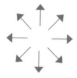

Activity Time!

Refer to Section 3—Activities.

CD-ROM

See Section 4 for directions.

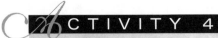
CTIVITY 4

CONSTRUCTING A HEALTH CARE REFERENCE LIST

Next, develop a reference list to present with your health care resume. A sample reference list, Figure 1-1-6, is shown as a guide. Carefully review this sample reference list, and then construct your own. Remove Activity 4 in Section 3. Use references who will speak well of you when they are asked about you by a prospective employer. If you have several references, select those who can talk about skills that relate to the specific health care job for which you are applying. Good references include former employers, instructors, friends, or neighbors who are well established in business or the health care industry. In general, family members or relatives should not be used as references. After you have drafted your reference list, show it to your instructor for evaluation. Key your reference list and save the final list on the same disk you used to store your resume. Print your final reference list on the same size and quality paper you used for your resume. Put your final reference list and your computer disk in your employment portfolio.

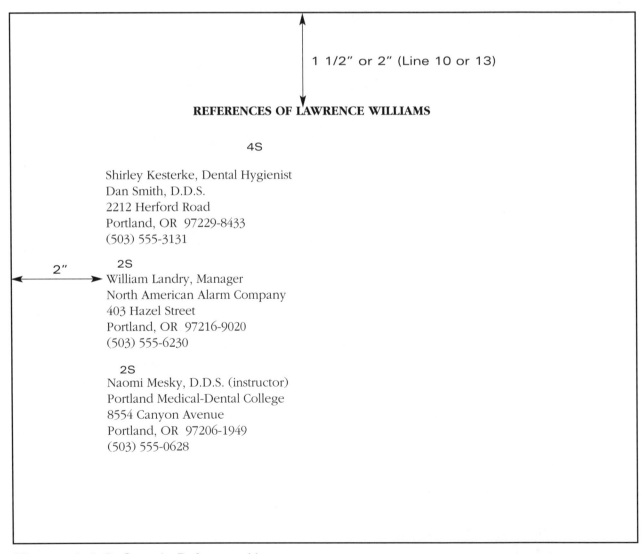

1 1/2" or 2" (Line 10 or 13)

REFERENCES OF LAWRENCE WILLIAMS

4S

Shirley Kesterke, Dental Hygienist
Dan Smith, D.D.S.
2212 Herford Road
Portland, OR 97229-8433
(503) 555-3131

2"   2S
William Landry, Manager
North American Alarm Company
403 Hazel Street
Portland, OR 97216-9020
(503) 555-6230

2S
Naomi Mesky, D.D.S. (instructor)
Portland Medical-Dental College
8554 Canyon Avenue
Portland, OR 97206-1949
(503) 555-0628

Figure 1-1-6 Sample Reference List

STEP 2
HEALTH CARE COVER LETTER

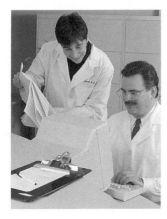

In this step you will find

- the definition of a health care cover letter (a letter of application).
- guidelines for writing and faxing a health care cover letter.
- three sample health care cover letters.
- an activity to help you write a health care cover letter.

WHAT IS A HEALTH CARE COVER LETTER?

A cover letter consists of a few simple paragraphs that state the position for which you are applying, your qualifications, and your request for an interview. It is important that this letter be clearly and concisely written, as it is usually the first contact you have with a prospective health care employer. You may also want to use a cover letter when presenting your resume in person. Remember the rewards of a good first impression. Always use a cover letter whenever you mail or fax a resume to a prospective health care employer.

HOW SHOULD YOU WRITE A HEALTH CARE COVER LETTER?

Use the following guidelines when writing a health care cover letter.

1. Address your letter to a specific person, if possible. If you do not have someone's name, call the health care facility and request the name of the human relations manager or supervisor in the service area in which you want to work. Some medical-related employment ads do not contain the name of a contact person, medical organization name, or street and city address. In some cases a fax number or P.O. box number replaces an address. See the sample cover letter, Figure 1-2-2, to see where to place a fax number.

   If you do not have an individual's name create a greeting by adding the word "manager" to the hiring department of an organization. For example, Dear Human Resource Manager, or Dear Human Relations Manager, or Dear Personnel Manager. You can also add the word manager to the service area that has the position you want. For example, Dear Medical Office Manager, or Dear Dental Office Receptionist Manager, or Dear Licensed Vocational Nurse Manager. (Read the sample cover letter, Figure 1-2-1, to see how a greeting was created.)

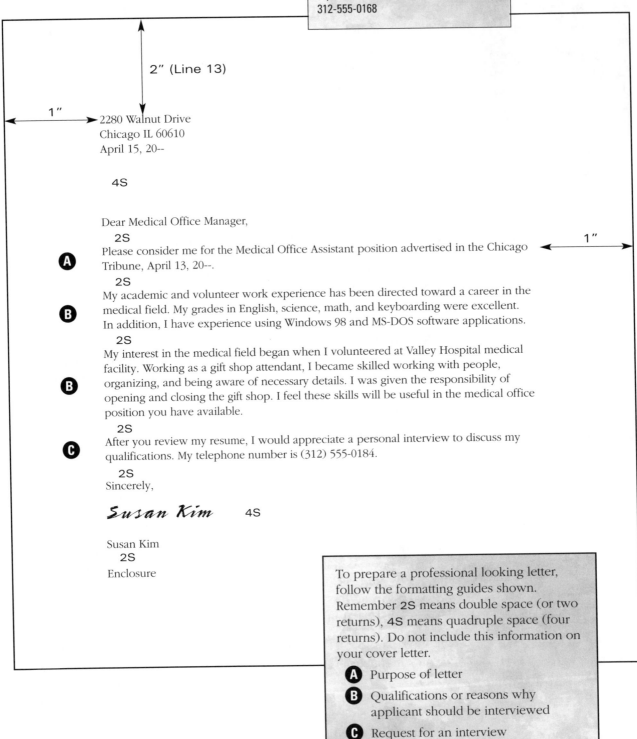

MEDICAL OFFICE ASSISTANT

P/T, No exp. necessary. Fast paced valley clinic. Team player. Fax resume to 312-555-0168

2" (Line 13)

1"

2280 Walnut Drive
Chicago IL 60610
April 15, 20--

4S

1"

Dear Medical Office Manager,

2S

A Please consider me for the Medical Office Assistant position advertised in the Chicago Tribune, April 13, 20--.

2S

B My academic and volunteer work experience has been directed toward a career in the medical field. My grades in English, science, math, and keyboarding were excellent. In addition, I have experience using Windows 98 and MS-DOS software applications.

2S

B My interest in the medical field began when I volunteered at Valley Hospital medical facility. Working as a gift shop attendant, I became skilled working with people, organizing, and being aware of necessary details. I was given the responsibility of opening and closing the gift shop. I feel these skills will be useful in the medical office position you have available.

2S

C After you review my resume, I would appreciate a personal interview to discuss my qualifications. My telephone number is (312) 555-0184.

2S

Sincerely,

Susan Kim   4S

Susan Kim

2S

Enclosure

To prepare a professional looking letter, follow the formatting guides shown. Remember **2S** means double space (or two returns), **4S** means quadruple space (four returns). Do not include this information on your cover letter.

A Purpose of letter

B Qualifications or reasons why applicant should be interviewed

C Request for an interview

Figure 1-2-1 Sample Cover Letter

2. State the purpose of your letter and the medical-related position for which you are applying.

3. State those qualifications that make you well suited for the health care position.

4. Request an interview.

5. Sign your letter before sending.

Your health care cover letter should be brief, clear, and carefully written. Proofread your letter for content. Have someone who is proficient in grammar edit your letter for correct spelling, punctuation, and grammar. *Remember:* any error in your cover letter will reflect poorly on you. Be sure to include a copy of your resume with each cover letter. Include any other requested information, such as samples of work.

Content of a Health Care Cover Letter

The content of a cover letter varies considerably depending upon the health care position you are seeking. Your health care cover letter paragraphs should include the following.

1. **Opening paragraph.** State why you are writing, the name of the health care position for which you are applying, and how you learned of the opening. If you are responding to an ad, state the date and name of the newspaper in which you saw the ad.

2. **Middle paragraph.** State why you are interested in working for the medical organization and why you desire this type of work. Point out your qualifications, achievements, training, and interest in the health care field.

3. **Closing paragraph.** Refer to your resume and encourage action. Ask for an interview or end with a question that encourages a reply. Instead of a statement such as, "I will appreciate hearing from you in the future."—which does not draw action—you might say, "I will call you next week to determine when we might meet to discuss the health care job opening." or "Please call me at (123) 846-XXXX concerning an interview to discuss the health care opening."

Sample Cover Letters

Three sample health care cover letters are presented in this step. In the first cover letter, Figure 1-2-1, Susan Kim, who has no paid work experience, is applying for a part-time medical office position. Ester Diaz, a recent graduate, writes the second health care cover letter, Figure 1-2-2. She is responding to a medical employment ad for a nurse's aide position. The third health care cover letter, Figure 1-2-3, shows that Thomas Lewis has followed up a contact from Mrs. Mayo, the placement officer for Hayward Dental Assisting College, concerning a job lead. He is sending a resume and cover letter to Ms. Toshi Yukimura.

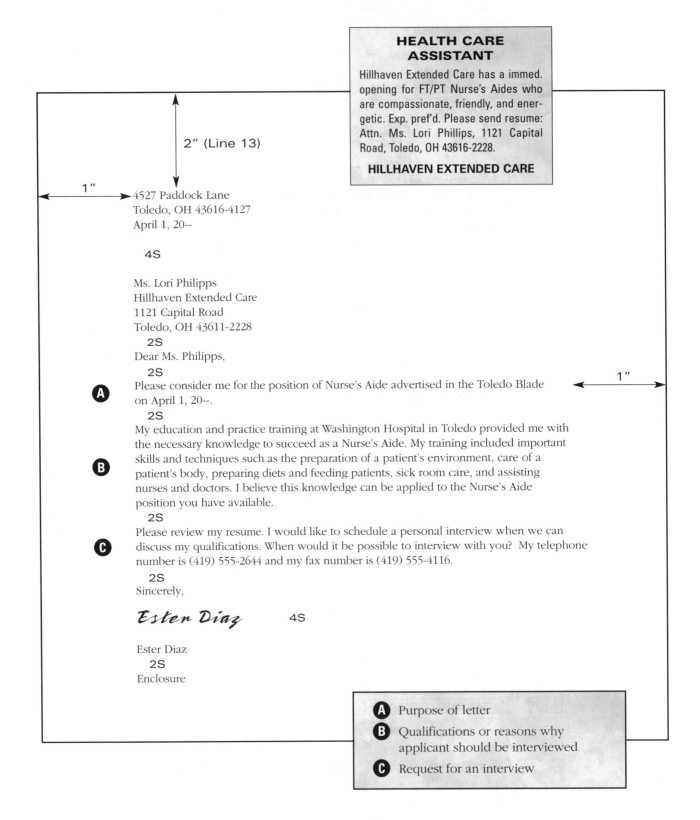

2" (Line 13)

1"

HEALTH CARE ASSISTANT

Hillhaven Extended Care has a immed. opening for FT/PT Nurse's Aides who are compassionate, friendly, and energetic. Exp. pref'd. Please send resume: Attn. Ms. Lori Phillips, 1121 Capital Road, Toledo, OH 43616-2228.

HILLHAVEN EXTENDED CARE

4527 Paddock Lane
Toledo, OH 43616-4127
April 1, 20--

4S

Ms. Lori Philipps
Hillhaven Extended Care
1121 Capital Road
Toledo, OH 43611-2228
2S
Dear Ms. Philipps,
2S
A Please consider me for the position of Nurse's Aide advertised in the Toledo Blade on April 1, 20--.
2S
B My education and practice training at Washington Hospital in Toledo provided me with the necessary knowledge to succeed as a Nurse's Aide. My training included important skills and techniques such as the preparation of a patient's environment, care of a patient's body, preparing diets and feeding patients, sick room care, and assisting nurses and doctors. I believe this knowledge can be applied to the Nurse's Aide position you have available.
2S
C Please review my resume. I would like to schedule a personal interview when we can discuss my qualifications. When would it be possible to interview with you? My telephone number is (419) 555-2644 and my fax number is (419) 555-4116.
2S
Sincerely,

Ester Diaz   4S

Ester Diaz
2S
Enclosure

1"

A Purpose of letter
B Qualifications or reasons why applicant should be interviewed
C Request for an interview

Figure 1-2-2 Sample Cover Letter

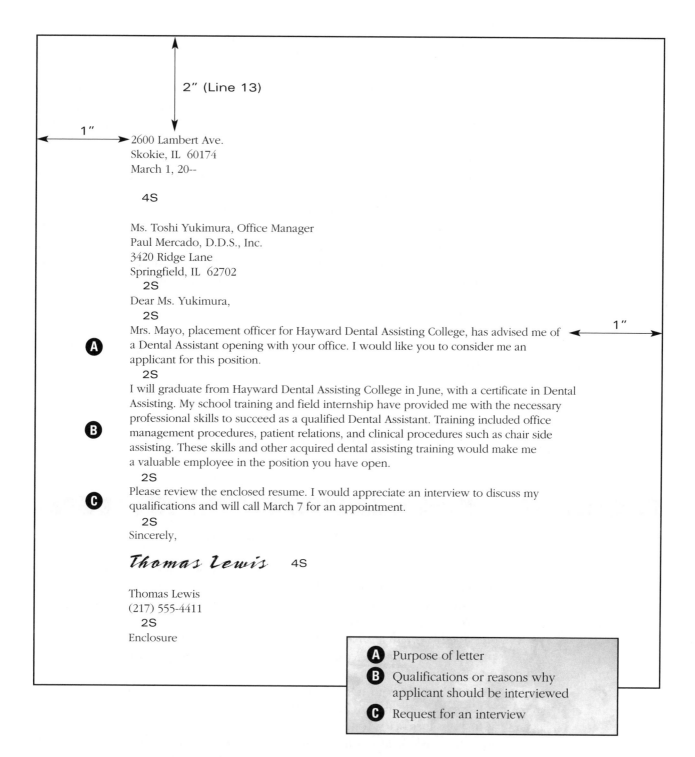

2" (Line 13)

1"

2600 Lambert Ave.
Skokie, IL 60174
March 1, 20--

4S

Ms. Toshi Yukimura, Office Manager
Paul Mercado, D.D.S., Inc.
3420 Ridge Lane
Springfield, IL 62702
    2S
Dear Ms. Yukimura,
    2S
A Mrs. Mayo, placement officer for Hayward Dental Assisting College, has advised me of
a Dental Assistant opening with your office. I would like you to consider me an
applicant for this position.
    2S

1"

B I will graduate from Hayward Dental Assisting College in June, with a certificate in Dental
Assisting. My school training and field internship have provided me with the necessary
professional skills to succeed as a qualified Dental Assistant. Training included office
management procedures, patient relations, and clinical procedures such as chair side
assisting. These skills and other acquired dental assisting training would make me
a valuable employee in the position you have open.
    2S

C Please review the enclosed resume. I would appreciate an interview to discuss my
qualifications and will call March 7 for an appointment.
    2S
Sincerely,

Thomas Lewis 4S

Thomas Lewis
(217) 555-4411
    2S
Enclosure

A Purpose of letter
B Qualifications or reasons why
   applicant should be interviewed
C Request for an interview

Figure 1-2-3 Sample Cover Letter

Read the health care employment ads, Figure 1-2-4, and notice that some do not ask for a cover letter. However, employers recognize that a cover letter shows a job applicant's extra effort and Susan, Ester, and Thomas all want jobs! The ad Susan is responding to uses a fax number instead of a name or address. Susan had two choices: she could send a cover letter without a greeting or add the title Manager to the medical office that has the job for which she is applying. She chose the latter. Ester sends her cover letter and resume to the person identified in the ad and Thomas sends his cover letter and resume to the person to whom his placement officer referred him.

Notice that all three job candidates state the purpose of their letter, list their medical job-related qualifications or reasons why they should be interviewed for the position, and request an interview. Notice that all candidates include their telephone number. You can also include your fax number or e-mail address. Try to make it as convenient as possible to be reached to establish a time for an interview.

Since Susan has no paid work experience, she uses her cover letter to explain how her school courses and volunteer work qualify her for the job. If you have little or no paid or volunteer work experience, use your school course medical-related training experience, including externship experience, and other relevant skills and interests to develop a winning cover letter.

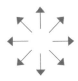

Activity Time!
Refer to Section 3—Activities.

CD-ROM
See Section 4 for directions.

ACTIVITY 5
WRITING A HEALTH CARE COVER LETTER

Review all of the newspaper medical-related employment ads in Figure 1-2-4. Select the job that is of most interest to you, and assume you have all of the qualifications. If you prefer, you may select an appropriate health care employment ad from your local newspaper. Then, remove the practice paper provided for Activity 5 in Section 3 and draft a cover letter. You may refer to the sample health care cover letters in this step when constructing your cover letter. Remember to look at the sample cover letters to decide where you want to include your telephone number with area code. Your fax and e-mail address may also be included. After you have drafted your cover letter show it to your instructor for evaluation. Then key your cover letter, saving it on the same disk used in this manual for your resume. Print your final cover letter on white 8 1/2" x 11" paper, the same quality used for your resume. Place your printed health care cover letter and computer disk in your employment portfolio for future reference.

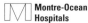
Figure 1-2-4 Newspaper Employment Ads

STEP 3
HEALTH CARE EMPLOYMENT APPLICATION

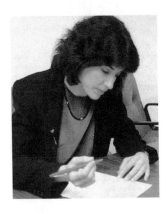

In this step you will find

- what health care employers want in an employment application.
- information needed to complete medical-related employment applications.
- a completed health care employment application to study.
- a choice of two blank health care employment applications to complete and use as references.

WHAT IS A HEALTH CARE EMPLOYMENT APPLICATION?

Most health care employers require applicants to complete an employment application. See Figure 1-3-1 for an example of a completed health care employment application. Employment applications are health care facility documents that give the employer facts about you that can be kept on file. These facts include basic information on your education, skills, work history, and references. Even if you have a resume and a scheduled interview, you will usually need to complete an employment application form. You should be prepared to complete the form when you go on an interview.

Be honest when you fill out a health care employment application. If you are hired and it is learned later that information on your application is untrue, you could be terminated for falsification of medical facility documents. For example, a claim on an application of a degree that someone doesn't have could cause that person to be fired for falsification of a health care organization document.

WHAT DO HEALTH CARE EMPLOYERS LOOK FOR IN AN EMPLOYMENT APPLICATION?

The information you provide and how well you present the information indicates to a health care employer the following:

1. **Your ability to follow instructions.** Have you carefully or carelessly filled out the employment application? Keep it neat. Your application may also indicate how well you can read and write.

2. **Your ability to hold a health care job.** There will be questions concerning your employment history. You may be asked to explain gaps in employment.

3. **Your achievements.** The employment application allows you to mention past accomplishments. Mention specifically those related to health care.

Follow directions.

If possible, use a ball point pen for neatness and effect. (blue or black ink).

Write out full school names, no abbreviations.

If you have no telephone, arrange to get a number where a message can be left. Write "(message)" next to the number.

Employees with little or no work experience should indicate "starting wage." Experienced employees should write "negotiable." Negotiable means that you would like to talk about the wage you have in mind.

Drawing a line shows you have read the statement or question and it does not apply to you.

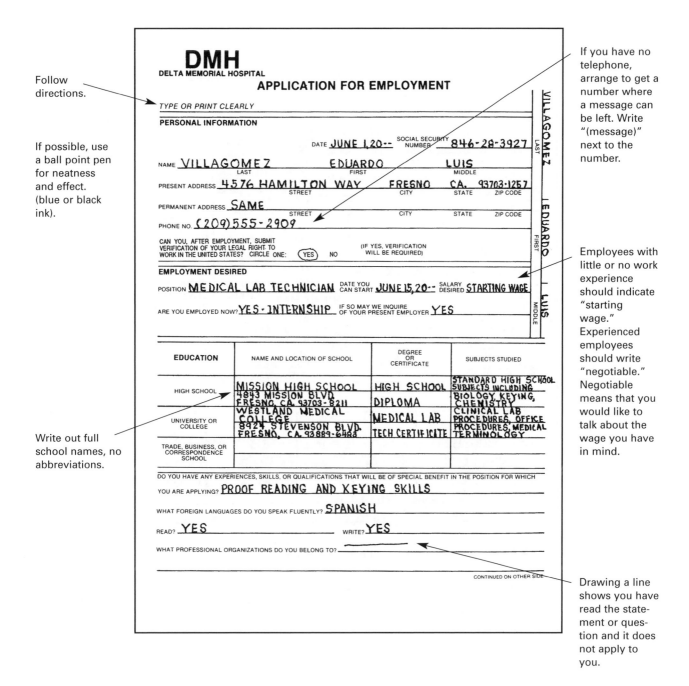

Figure 1-3-1 Sample Employment Application (Front)

WORK EXPERIENCE

List all present and past employment, including part-time or seasonal, beginning with the most recent.

Employer	Employment Dates and Salary	Describe the work you did in detail	Reason for leaving
Name RAVENWOOD HOSPITAL Address 4242 BLACOW RD. City FRESNO State CA. (209) Phone 555-1816 Supervisor MRS. R. POHLI	From: JAN., 20-- To: PRESENT Salary NONE	MEDICAL LAB TECH. COLLECT AND EXAMINE BLOOD, TISSUE AND FLUID SAMPLES. PREPARED STAIN SLIDES FOR MICROORGANISMS AND ANALYZE CHEMICAL COMPONENTS.	INTERNSHIP
Name ROUND TABLE PIZZA Address 296 DURHAM RD. City FRESNO State CA. (209) Phone 555-4155 Supervisor JOHN ROBERTS	From: SEPT 20-- To: JAN, 20-- Salary $6.25	COUNTER PERSON CASHIER, SERVE CUSTOMERS, GENERAL MAINTENANCE	TO PURSUE A CAREER POSITION
Name FRESNO MAIN LIBRARY Address 9846 PASEO PADRE City FRESNO State CA. (209) Phone 555-6132 Supervisor DONALD CONLEY	From: JUNE 20-- To: AUG, 20-- Salary MINIMUM WAGE	LIBRARY ASSISTANT STACKING AND FILING BOOKS. CODING LIBRARY MATERIALS	END OF SUMMER EMPLOYMENT PROGRAM
Name MERCY HOSPITAL Address 312 BALBOA DR. City FRESNO State CA. (209) Phone 555-8300 Supervisor DANA WALSH	From: JUNE, 20-- To: AUG, 20-- Salary NONE	VOLUNTEER ASSISTANT, GIFT SHOP. SERVE CUSTOMERS, GENERAL MAINTENANCE	RETURN TO SCHOOL

Keep your reasons for leaving past jobs positive. They should sound good.

REFERENCES: GIVE BELOW THE NAMES OF THREE PERSONS NOT RELATED TO YOU, WHOM YOU HAVE KNOWN AT LEAST ONE YEAR.

NAME	ADDRESS	BUSINESS	YEARS ACQUAINTED
1 MRS. ROBERT POHLI	4242 BLACOW RD. FRESNO CA 93703-1245	RAVENWOOD HOSP. FRESNO CA	6 MONTHS INTERNSHIP
2 MR. JOHN ROBERTS	296 DURHAM RD. FRESNO, CA 93703-6844	ROUND TABLE (MANAGER)	2½ YEARS
3 MR. DONALD CONLEY	3846 PASEO PADRE FRESNO, CA. 93889	FRESNO MAIN LIBRARY FRESNO, CA	1 YEAR

IN CASE OF EMERGENCY NOTIFY MRS. ANNA VILLAGOMEZ
NAME

8233 FREMONT AVE., FRESNO, CA. 93703   (209) 555-3838
ADDRESS   PHONE NO.

I AUTHORIZE INVESTIGATION OF ALL STATEMENTS CONTAINED IN THIS APPLICATION. I UNDERSTAND THAT MISREPRESENTATION OR OMISSION OF FACTS CALLED FOR IS CAUSE FOR DISMISSAL. FURTHER, I UNDERSTAND AND AGREE THAT MY EMPLOYMENT IS FOR NO DEFINITE PERIOD AND MAY, REGARDLESS OF THE DATE OF PAYMENT OF MY WAGES AND SALARY, BE TERMINATED AT ANY TIME WITHOUT ANY PREVIOUS NOTICE.

DATE June 1, 20--   SIGNATURE Eduardo L. Villagomez

When signing your application use your full name. Never use a nickname.

Figure 1-3-1 Sample Employment Application (Back)

4. **Your thoroughness.** Did you answer all the questions on the employment application? Don't leave blanks. Drawing a line or placing N/A (not applicable) shows the employer you have read the question and it does not apply to you.

Completing a health care employment application does not automatically ensure an interview. The outcome could depend on how well you completed the employment application. *Remember:* always include a copy of your resume with your employment application.

Completing a Health Care Employment Application

Gather the information and materials needed to complete your medical-related employment application. Much of the information you are seeking is on your resume. Make sure you have the following when completing a health care employment application.

1. Two pens (blue or black ink), two pencils, an eraser, paper clips

2. Your current and previous addresses and Social Security number

3. Education information, usually from high school to present. Give names and addresses of schools, the diplomas or degrees you earned, and the dates you attended each institution. Indicate any subjects, particularly those relating to health care, in which you excelled.

4. Work records. Be able to provide the names, addresses, and phone numbers of past employers; the dates of employment; job responsibilities; the wages earned; the names of your supervisors; and your reasons for leaving each job. Keep your reasons for leaving a job positive. Include military experience (if any) and volunteer work.

5. List of your health care, medical business, and machine operation skills

6. Names of certificates, licenses, professional organizations, and other medical-related documents, honors, and achievements that could give you an advantage over other applicants

7. A list of references that shows names, job titles, health care facility names and company names, addresses, and telephone numbers

8. Copies of your resume. Remember to attach your resume to any completed employment application with a paper clip.

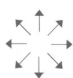

Activity Time!
Refer to Section 3—Activities.

ACTIVITY 6
COMPLETING A HEALTH CARE EMPLOYMENT APPLICATION

Before you begin, read the completed sample application, Figure 1-3-1, in this step. Then, gather the information and materials noted earlier in this section. Remove Activity 6 in Section 3 and complete one of two blank health care employment applications. First determine what health care job you are seeking. The key is to think of a health care job title that you are interested in or qualified for in the near future. If necessary you can reference job titles in *The Dictionary of Occupational Titles* that can be found in your library or online at http://www.oalj.dol.gov/libdot.htm. You can also access the *Occupational Outlook Handbook* at http://www.stats.bls.gov/oco/home.htm. The Delta Memorial Hospital and Pacific Medical Center are very large medical organizations; you need to be specific. They have many career opportunities, including the health care position you want. When you have completed your employment application to your satisfaction, show it to your instructor for evaluation. Then place your completed employment application in your employment portfolio. Use it as a reference when completing application forms for health care jobs.

STEP 4
FINDING AND RESEARCHING A HEALTH CARE JOB AND FACILITY

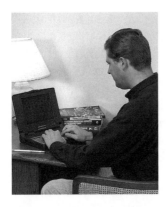

In this step you will find

- the definition of a job lead.
- ten sources of health care job leads.
- a method for recording health care job leads and contacts.
- a method for researching a health care job and facility.

WHAT IS A JOB LEAD?

A job lead is a contact that may direct you to a job opening. A job lead in health care may be found

- in a newspaper or professional medical journal that lists job openings.
- by talking to someone who might know about a health care job opening.
- by visiting a health care facility that may have a job opening.
- by contacting employment agencies.
- by exploring internet health care employment Web sites.

You need to find and act on as many health care job leads as possible. The time and effort you spend looking for a job represents a considerable investment in your future. Finding the right job takes time, organization, and requires a commitment.

There are many ways to get a health care job other than just submitting an application. In fact, the more contacts you make in the health care field, the better your chances of finding employment. Job leads can give you a good idea of what kind of medical-related work is available. When you pursue job leads, different people get to know you and your medical career goals.

HOW CAN I FIND HEALTH CARE JOB LEADS?

Following is a list of ten sources of health care job leads that you can use. Can you think of any others?

Job Lead 1: School Career Center or Placement Office. School career centers and placement offices are excellent sources for health care job leads. Contact your school career center and/or placement office for medical-related job opportunities. Placement counselors may not only have a health care job lead for you but may offer other services such, as assisting you in resume writing, and keying and printing a resume. You will be provided with an employment application to complete and file with your school career center and/or placement office. Your placement counselor will contact employers and provide a list of health care job openings. Ask the employment counselor to set up an interview for you.

Job Lead 2: Market Survey. Use the Yellow Pages to make a list of medical offices, dental offices, hospitals, clinics, and laboratories in your area. Telephone each health care facility and ask to talk with the personnel manager or office manager.

Rather than presenting yourself as a job seeker, say something like, "I am really interested in working as a medical assistant (limited scope X-ray technician, surgical technologist, or whatever) when I finish my training. I would like to find out about jobs in this field. Can you tell me about the work that is done here, and how a person like myself could get started in this field?"

Ask if you could visit the workplace. This method allows you to learn about health care employment possibilities even though there may be no job openings. This technique is often referred to as an "informational interview." Most people enjoy talking about their work and giving advice to a good listener. Furthermore, they may remember you when there is a job opening.

Job Lead 3: Associations. Your local library has a list of established professional medical associations. These associations can help you become familiar with the training and education required for a specific health care job. They are important sources of immediate job opportunities because they often publish informative magazines that include employment want ads. Your polite letter to the president of an association's local chapter might be answered with, "Come visit us anytime!" Ask your librarian for assistance in locating these publications. Also, look in the Yellow Pages under the heading "Associations."

Job Lead 4: Networking. Some health care jobs are never advertised. Make an effort to tell your friends, relatives, people you meet in the health care field, and acquaintances that you want a job in health care. People you see in places you go everyday may just have a lead—you have to let them know you want a job in health care! If possible, give people who offer to help you a copy of your completed resume. Your resume will serve as a constant reminder that you are looking for a health care position.

Job Lead 5: Newspaper Employment Ads. Carefully read the health care help-wanted ads in your local newspaper. Follow up on those health care employment ads that look promising. Do not just look for ads with a special title such as Medical Assistant, as there may be other jobs advertised where you could use your skills and talents. Send a cover letter and resume when responding to an employment ad.

Job Lead 6: Private Employment Agencies. Private employment agencies that specialize in handling health care personnel are listed under "Employment Agencies" in the Yellow Pages. Contact them for a screening and an interview. Give them a copy of your resume. Many job openings are placed with private employment agencies rather than listed in newspaper want ads.

Private employment agencies may provide the job seeker with health care employment. They also provide job leads, career counseling, assistance in resume writing, and interview techniques. Deal only with an employment agency that has a good reputation. Some employment agencies may charge you a fee for their services; others charge the employer with whom they found you a job. Normally the employment agency will want you to sign an employment contract. Be sure to agree to the requirements and cost, if any, of the contract before signing.

Job Lead 7: Temporary Employment Agencies. Temporary employment agencies are listed under "Employment" or "Employment—Temporary" in the Yellow Pages. You may want a temporary health care job simply to get work experience. Temporary jobs can last from a few hours to several months. Many health care employers need extra help for special projects and during vacations or employee leaves of absence. Temporary employment may lead to a permanent job. These temporary health care experiences can help in making sound medical career employment decisions.

Job Lead 8: State Employment Office. Look in your telephone directory for the phone number of your state employment office, which has health care career information and job-hunting tips. Call them and ask about their employment workshops and their procedures for assisting you in your job search. Visit your state employment office and check the medical-related job openings that are posted or filed. Fill out an application and set up an interview with a counselor. The counselor will match your qualifications to current health care job openings. Your local state employment office can also advise you of state civil service health care employment opportunities.

Job Lead 9: U.S. Civil Service Employment Office. Look in your telephone directory for the nearest United States Federal Civil Service Employment Office. This type of employment office is generally located in large cities. Call or visit this office and ask what government health care jobs are available. Ask what the procedures are for getting a job in health care with the United States Federal Civil Service. Be prepared to take the Civil Service Test in order to earn a government service rating. Write for employment opportunities with the U.S. Civil Service, U.S. Office of Personnel Management, 1900 E Street NW, Washington, DC 20415-0001, or check their Web site at http://www.opm.gov. It is possible to inquire directly to a Federal medical facility such as a Veteran's Administration (V.A.) hospital for employment.

Job Lead 10: Your Internet Job Search. Many health care facilities have established Web sites on the Internet. These sites often contain job ads and other information on current job openings. Many state and federal agencies also post job openings on the Internet. If you need help using the Internet or locating health care Web sites, go to your school career office or public library. Their staff can show you how to research health care job openings through their Internet provider.

Here are Internet Web sites of some health care employment resources that you can explore for health care job opportunities and tips for gaining employment.

America's Job Bank	http://www.ajb.dni.us/
Career Mosaic	http://www.careermosaic.com/
Career Builder	http://www.careerbuilder.com/
Catapult	http://www.jobweb.org/catapult/
JobBank USA	http://www.jobbankusa.com/
JobWeb	http://www.jobweb.org/
Monster.com	http://www.monster.com/

Here are some Internet search engines to locate health care job and employer Web sites.

Alta Visa	http://www.altavista.com/
Excite	http://www.excite.com/
Lycos	http://www.lycos.com/
Yahoo	http://www.yahoo.com/

Researching a Health Care Job

If you are interested in a particular health care job title and want to learn more about it, talk to people who do that kind of work. Ask them what health care duties are performed, what skills are required, and what the medical career opportunities are.

To research health care job titles check with your school library, career center, placement office, or counselor; local library; or bookstore for comprehensive resources that contain health care job descriptions. A job description is a written report defining specific job duties and listing the minimum qualifications for a job. A job description will give you a clear picture of what is expected of that medical-related job. Also at these facilities you can find books listing medical associations. Contact medical associations to find out what health care openings are available.

You will find books that include general health care job descriptions as well job descriptions for specific medical career areas, such as a clinical medical technician, pharmacy technician, medical office manager, dental assistant, and surgical technologist. Two books that will help you get started learning about specific jobs are

1. *Dictionary of Occupational Titles* published by the U.S. Department of Labor. This handbook briefly describes every known occupation in the U.S.

2. *Occupational Outlook Handbook* published by the U.S. Department of Labor. This handbook gives complete descriptions of major occupations.

You should know the answers to the following questions about a health care job before you go for an interview.

1. What skills, education, and experience are required for this job?

2. What are the job duties?

Researching a Health Care Facility

To find out more about a specific health care facility you can

- talk to people who work at the medical facility. Ask them what services the health care facility provides, and what it is like to work there.

- write or call the medical facility for information. Say you are interested in learning about the services they provide. Tell them that you want to learn how it got started, and what important things have happened in the medical facility to improve its services.

- use the Internet. Check the health care facility Web site for information on its mission, philosophy, and services.

- go to a large bookstore and look in the career section for books that list names of medical facilities, addresses, telephone numbers, and Web sites.

- go to the library to see if there are any books, newspapers, or magazine articles about the health care facility. If the facility is publicly owned and local, the library may also have a copy of the annual report for you to examine. Ask the reference librarian to help you. Some examples that may help you research a publicly owned health care facility include:

  Publications:
  Barron's
  Wall Street Journal
  Value Line Investment Survey
  Standard & Poor's Stock Reports
  Dunn & Bradstreet
  Reader's Guide to Periodical Literature

  Magazines:
  Forbes
  Fortune
  Business Week
  Time

You should know as much about a health care facility as you can before you send out a resume or go for an interview. Answers to two questions give the most important information for you to know.

1. What services does this health care facility provide?

2. What kinds of health care jobs does it have?

Other questions also help you become informed. How old is the health care facility? In what cities does this health care organization have facilities? What is the size of this medical organization? Is it growing or shrinking in number of employees? Who are this medical organization's competitors? (Competitors are health care facilities that provide the same type of services.)

Important: Your research should lead to you having other questions about the health care facility. After you have all of the above questions answered about the medical organization, think of others that you would like answered. These are questions you may want to ask at a health care job interview.

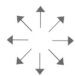

Activity Time!
Refer to Section 3—Activities.

CD-ROM
See Section 4 for directions.

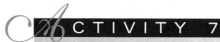

CTIVITY 7
FINDING HEALTH CARE JOB LEADS

Carefully examine each type of health care job lead presented in this step. Decide which leads you wish to pursue. For each health care lead, record the name of your contact; the phone number, fax, and e-mail if available; the address; and any notes you may have on your conversation with them. Remove the forms provided in Section 3 for Activity 7. Keeping track of your health care contacts during your job search gives an accurate record of where you applied for a job and where you want to follow up. When you have completed your job leads to your satisfaction, show them to your instructor for evaluation. Place all vital job lead information in your employment portfolio.

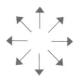

Activity Time!
Refer to Section 3—Activities.

CTIVITY 8
RESEARCHING A HEALTH CARE FACILITY

A visit to your school or local library will likely be necessary to complete this activity. Note the publications and magazines that are available for research in this step. Also ask the reference librarian for other research suggestions. Remove Activity 8 in Section 3. Select and research one to three health care facilities for this activity. Record your answers to the research questions on the health care facilities you selected. When you have completed your research paper to your satisfaction, show it to your instructor for evaluation. Then place it in your employment portfolio as a guide for researching a health care facility for a future job.

STEP 5
HOW TO PREPARE FOR A HEALTH CARE INTERVIEW

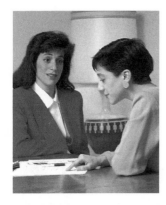

In this step you will find

- a discussion about personal preparation and why it is important.
- the twelve most common interview questions and their appropriate responses.
- a writing exercise to help you answer the twelve common interview questions.
- a list of questions you should consider concerning the job opening and the health care facility.
- a checklist to help you prepare for a health care interview.

WHY IS PERSONAL PREPARATION IMPORTANT?

Congratulations, you have an interview. Your hard work has paid off. Your letter and resume have convinced a prospective employer to interview you for a health care position. Now you need to prepare yourself for a successful job interview. Personal preparation for an interview is important. Being well prepared before the interview increases your self-confidence. Making a good first impression on the interviewer helps the interviewer determine where you will best fit in the health care facility.

Your goals at that interview will be to learn more about the job, convince the employer you are the right person for the job, and gather enough information about the health care facility and job to determine if you want the position, if it is offered.

WHAT TO DO BEFORE A HEALTH CARE INTERVIEW

Find out as much as you can about the health care facility. If you did not research the facility before responding to a job lead, you should do so before you have your interview. Reread the section on researching a company in Section 1, Step 4 and follow the guidelines there. At a minimum, you should know what the health care facility does, what services it offers, the kinds of jobs it provides, and the positions that are available. You may also want to find out how long the facility has been in business, the size of the facility (is it growing or shrinking in number of employees and services?), in what cities it has other health care facilities, the prospects for the future, the facility's public image, and its competitors. You will make a great impression in the interview if you relate what you know about the health care facility. You should tell what impresses you about the facility and what you find most interesting.

Be organized. You now have your employment portfolio. You should bring all the material you need for the health care interview in it to the interview. This includes another copy of your resume, your cover letter, your reference list, and a completed employment application. Organize this material and any other information you need in your employment portfolio. You'll also want to arrive on time and have a nice appearance. Before the interview, review and use Figure 1-5-1, the Interview Checklist. It will help you make a good impression at the interview.

Think about questions you'll be asked and how to answer them. You may be asked to provide more detail on information provided in your resume or application. There are many possible questions that may be asked during a health care interview. Of these, the twelve questions that follow— or some variation of them—are among the most common. Prepare yourself for your own interview by reading these questions and their suggested answers. Keep in mind the suggested answers are examples of good business-like responses. Consider what makes each response a good one. Whenever

Interview Checklist

Post and read this checklist one week before the interview to remind yourself what you need to do. Reread it the night before the interview. Place a check mark (✓) beside each item as you complete it.

When Interview Is Scheduled

☐ Review your research or research the health care facility.

☐ Prepare a card with the time and place of the interview and the name of the interviewer. Mark the date and time in your calendar.

☐ Get directions to location. A practice run may be helpful.

Day Before the Interview

● **Gather the following supplies in your Employment Portfolio or brief case:**

☐ Two pens and two pencils for filling out forms at the interview

☐ Money for parking, lunch, etc.

☐ Resume

☐ Completed employment application from Step 3. Use it as a reference when completing the company's employment application.

☐ Samples of your work (keyboarding samples, diagrams, etc.)

☐ Military records

☐ Social Security number

☐ Diplomas and special training certificates

☐ Licenses—driver's license or other special licenses

☐ Reference letters or list

☐ Other papers or materials that will help you obtain employment

● **Plan your appearance:**

☐ Check to see if you need a hair cut.

☐ Lay out clothes you are to wear. Check that they are clean, mended, pressed, and an appropriate style.

☐ Polish shoes

Day of the Interview

● **Check your appearance:**

☐ Hair is washed and styled.

☐ Body is bathed; deodorant is used.

☐ Make-up, jewelry, and perfume or after-shave lotion is not used excessively.

☐ Fingernails are trimmed and clean.

☐ Teeth are clean; breath is fresh.

Going to the Interview

☐ Leave for the interview early. Take the card with the directions and phone number with you.

☐ Go alone to the interview.

☐ Be polite in the outer office.

☐ Know the name(s) and title(s) of the person(s) who will interview you.

☐ Allow enough time for the interview.

Figure 1-5-1 Interview Checklist

you have an interview, read these questions with a specific health care facility and job in mind. Then prepare and *practice, practice, practice* your answers until you feel comfortable and sound confident.

THE TWELVE MOST COMMON INTERVIEW QUESTIONS

1. **In what type of health care position are you most interested?**

   When you respond to this question, be specific. State the type of health care job you want and the education and applicable skills you have.

   "Because I am good at keying, filing, scheduling appointments, and all jobs related to medical office work, I would be an excellent medical receptionist."

   "I am experienced in the care and use of EKG equipment and in preparing patients for the EKG series. I am familiar with EKG safety precautions, and all other work related to being an EKG technician."

2. **Why do you want to leave your current job? or Why did you leave your last job?**

   When you respond to this question, be honest but positive about why you want to leave your current job or left your last job. If you were fired from a job, this may be a difficult question. Keep in mind that most employers are willing to give an applicant a chance if it can be determined that the person understands why they lost their job and is trying to improve. Always be honest. You will lose your chance of obtaining a health care job if it is discovered that you lied during the interview. See Section 2, Step 4, Special Circumstances: When You Must Leave a Health Care Job, for more guidance on answering this question when you are fired or laid off.

   "While I enjoy working for my current health care facility, I want a more responsible and challenging job position."

   "I realize that I do not enjoy working at a desk all day. I am interested in pursuing a career in helping people with health problems."

   "My health care facility eliminated my job in a downsizing."

3. **What pay do you expect?**

   Know what the range is for the position you want before the interview. You may find this out from the health care facilities employment office or from the original job lead. The lead may also include some clues to the salary range. "Beginners Welcome" suggests a salary range at the low end of the range. If no salary information is available, find out what the salary range is for that type of health care work. If you do not know what the range is, ask. You may also ask if the salary is negotiable.

   "Considering my experience, what is the hourly pay range for this job?"

   "I understand that the salary range for this position is $15–$20,000. Based on the responsibilities you've described and my experience, I believe $20–$25,000 would be appropriate."

4. **Why do you want to work for our health care facility?**

Obtain information about the facility before attending the interview. To answer this question you will want to gather as much positive feedback about the health care facility as you can. If possible obtain information about the type of health services rendered, working conditions, work environment, career opportunities, and responsiveness to patients' needs. This information might come from people who work for the health care employer, past employees, patients who use its services, persons who are familiar with the health care industry, and your own observation and judgment. Your efforts will show that you are seriously interested in working for the health care facility. This information will allow you to discuss the health care facility intelligently. Note the following responses:

"My friends (or people you know who work for the health care facility) have commented to me on your excellent reputation for patient care. My goal is to work for a hospital that shows this kind of concern for its patients."

"Your office is well known for the competent medical care it gives your patients. I would like to work for a medical office with such a fine reputation."

"I enjoy working with and helping people. The challenge of this position is exciting."

5. **Have you had any serious illness or injury that might prevent you from performing your duties in this position?**

The response to this question is easy if there has been no problem. However, if in the past you had a medical problem or injury, be prepared to show a clearance slip from your physician. The clearance slip should state that you are physically able to perform the job you are seeking. If you have no physical problem, you might say:

"No, I am in excellent health and can perform all duties required as a dental assistant."

However, if you had a problem in the past, the following answer would be appropriate:

"At this time, I can perform all of the duties of a surgical technologist. My medical problem in the past has been corrected and here is my physician's clearance slip."

6. **Do you have references?**

Your ability to get good references says a great deal about you. A reference (or recommendation) is generally a positively written series of statements about your character, attitude, skills, and abilities. Most reference checking is done by phone. Be prepared to hand over a reference list like the one shown in this manual. If you have a reference letter, be prepared to discuss that as well. An example of a reference letter is shown in Section 2, Step 3, Figure 2-3-1.

"Here is my reference list. Jane Smith is very familiar with my word-processing skills. She told me to tell you that the best time to reach her by phone is before noon."

7. What did you like *best* or *least* about your last job?

Do not downgrade previous employers or supervisors. Always remain positive about your last job. Tell what general and specific things you liked most. You might say something like:

"There were many things I liked about my last job. The two most important items were the people I worked with and my specific job duties."

Try not to respond to things you did not like about your last job.

8. Are you looking for a permanent or temporary job? Do you want full-time or part-time work?

The time structure of health care jobs may be temporary part time, temporary full time, permanent part time, or permanent full time. A temporary part-time job may involve a few hours of work per week, or the job may last only one month during the year. A temporary full-time job may involve daily work for a week, month, or half a year.

A permanent part-time job would be fewer than 35 hours a week for a year or more of employment. A permanent full-time job would involve the regular 40-hour week with vacations and holidays. Remember, you gain experience with a temporary or permanent part-time job. This experience may lead to a permanent full-time job with the same health care facility. Employers are more inclined to hire experienced help from within the health care facility than they are to hire someone from the outside. If you really want to work within a particular health care facility try to be flexible. You might say something like:

"At this time I am interested in a permanent full-time position, but if none are available I would agree to a part-time job until a full-time position becomes available."

9. Tell me something about yourself. Why do you think we should hire you for this job?

Keep your answer on a professional level. In other words, discuss only those traits that relate to the health care job. Mention your educational background, internships, work experience, and any skills, interests, and hobbies you have that would make you the best choice for the job.

"I can bring to the job the following: excellent accounting skills, accurate keying at 60 words a minute, accurate 10-key operation, excellent patient relations skills, and excellent nursing assistant skills, such as bed changes, bathing, feeding, and general hygiene."

10. How well do you work under pressure?

Almost all jobs require a worker to meet some deadlines. To give a positive answer to this question you might say,

"My present work requires me to meet deadlines. I have excellent time management and organizational skills to meet these deadlines without undue pressure."

11. What are your strengths and weaknesses?

Describe your strengths. This shows confidence and a positive attitude. If possible, do not discuss any weakness you might have. Sell yourself;

modesty will not win you a job. Be prepared to back up statements with past examples. Possible strengths might be:

"I learn new skills quickly. On my last job I became proficient in Microsoft Word and front office procedures within a week."

"I work well under pressure. With Baxter Medical I never missed a monthly billing deadline."

"I am thorough with my assignments. My proofreading skills are excellent."

If it is necessary to describe a weakness, use the suggestion described here or a similar one. Be prepared to turn a weakness into strength. For example:

"I'm a perfectionist. I do not feel comfortable handing over a job that is less than the best I can do—even if it means working on it on my own time."

Or, "Some co-workers think I am too organized. But I find it really saves time in the long run if I budget time each day for part of a big job so I meet the deadline."

12. **What are your short-term and long-term employment goals?**

A safe short-term goal answer might be:

"My goal is to become a productive employee in a short period of time. I am anxious to learn all I can about Respiratory Therapy and the health care field."

A safe long-term goal answer might be:

"My long-term goal is to become a true professional and team member as a Respiratory Therapist. In addition I would like to obtain my Registered Respiratory Therapist (RRT) Credential."

There are, of course, hundreds of potential questions. Some other common interview questions include:

Tell me about your education.

Tell me about an achievement of which you are most proud.

Tell me about a time when you encountered a difficult situation. What happened and how did you handle it?

Take each question as an opportunity to talk about your skills and strengths and to learn more about the requirements of the job for which you are applying.

GETTING THE RIGHT ANSWERS TO THE RIGHT QUESTIONS

Generally speaking, you should not start a discussion about salary or wages. Let the interviewer initiate this conversation. Job seekers should not ask certain questions during an interview because they may seem inappropriate or insensitive. For example: How much will I make? What days do I get off? How much vacation time do I get? How many paid holidays do I get? How much sick leave do I get? These questions are self-serving. More concern is shown for *getting out of work* than for *getting a job*. Although the questions are important, they usually will be answered before you need to ask. This kind of information is a normal part of any serious interview.

Therefore, a very important part of the interview process is asking the *right questions* in the *right way* and at the *right time*. By researching the health care facility thoroughly, you will be prepared to ask a number of appropriate questions that could determine whether you would in fact enjoy the type of work the facility has to offer. Many people have accepted job offers only to find that the work, the health care facility, and the services were not what they expected. These people did not adequately research the employer nor ask the right questions at the interview.

Think about the Questions You Want to Ask

An interview is a two-way process and you also want to find out information about the job, working conditions, and growth opportunities with the health care facility. Employers expect the right answers from you, and you should expect the right answers from them. Your work represents one of the most time-consuming aspects of your life. Decisions about job offers should always be made with care and research. Good decisions will lead to job satisfaction. This will add greatly to the success of your health care career.

There are several important questions you will want answered *before* accepting a job offer. The employment questions that follow are divided into two categories: those regarding you and the job opening, and those regarding you and the health care facility. Asking good questions about the job opening and the health care facility indicates to the employer that you are an intelligent, informed candidate for the position. More importantly, the answers to these questions may give you the necessary information to make a very important lifetime decision—accepting a health care job you will like. These questions and their answers will come from your *research* of the company, your *observation* of the workplace, *information* provided during the interview, and any *questions* you ask during the interview.

You and the Job Opening

- Why is there a job opening?
- Where have others who have held this job been reassigned within the health care facility?
- When might a person expect to be promoted?
- How and when is a new employee to be evaluated?
- Does the employee evaluation system seem fair?
- Is the health care position challenging or will it be boring work as time goes on?
- What training can a new employee expect?
- Will there be an employee probationary period (a trial period before becoming a permanent employee)?
- Is the physical work environment clean, well decorated, and properly maintained?

● Are co-workers compatible with you in age and experience?

Add any other questions that you would like to have answered.

_____

_____

You and the Health Care Facility

● How does the facility's employee wage and benefit package compare with others in the same industry?

● Can a new employee expect regular wage increases?

● What is the employee turnover rate at this facility?

● What are some of the health care facility's new services?

● What is the employer's reputation in the community and in the industry?

● How are health services offered by the organization rated in the field?

● How will the employer's rules and regulations affect you?

● How will the employer's work expectations and work hours affect your private life?

Add any other questions that you would like to have answered.

_____

_____

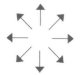

Activity Time!
Refer to Section 3—Activities.

Refer to Section 3—Activities.

CTIVITY 9

ANSWERING INTERVIEW QUESTIONS

To begin this exercise, identify a specific job at a specific health care facility for which you would like to interview. You may use one of the job leads you identified in Step 4 or the health care facility you wrote a cover letter to in Step 2. Then remove the worksheets for Activity 9 in Section 3. Write your answers to the twelve most common interview questions. You may refer to the answers provided in this manual when writing your answers.

When you have answered the questions to your satisfaction, show them to your instructor for evaluation. Then work in groups of two or three. Have one person act as the interviewer and ask each question. Answer them with your written replies. Have the interviewer and a third person give you their impressions, then switch roles. If you practice answering the questions before you attend the actual interview, your confidence will definitely increase. Put your answers to the interview questions with any changes or comments suggested by your evaluators and instructor in your employment portfolio.

STEP 6
DURING THE HEALTH CARE INTERVIEW

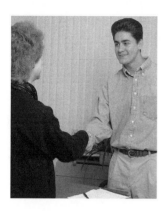

In this step you will find

- a general description of a health care interview.
- "do's and don'ts" for health care interviews.
- a case study of a model health care interview.
- questions about the model health care interview.

THE HEALTH CARE INTERVIEW

The interview is your chance to sell yourself. You must give the impression that you have the skills necessary for the health care job you are seeking, that you are dependable, and that you get along well with people. Knowing what to do and what not to do during the interview ensures confidence and success. Be aware that most health care interviews usually contain the following four stages.

1. introduction (what the health care position is about)

2. questions about you and your qualification

3. questions from you about the job, health care facility, etc.

4. closing remarks

Stage 1: Introduction. Start your interview like a winner. Have a good attitude. Your first greeting to the interviewer is critical to your being hired. Be enthusiastic. Frequently interviewers make hiring decisions based on first impressions. Make a positive first impression by smiling and establishing eye contact with the interviewer when you introduce yourself. Extend a firm handshake, and say, "Hello, Mrs. Sutton, I am Nancy Karr." Practice this technique with a family member or friend.

Stage 2: Questions about you. During the question stage, the employer will be leading the interview. The interviewer will be asking questions such as, "Why should we hire you?" or "Why do you want to work for this health care facility?" Listen carefully. Answer all questions in a brief, concise manner. Relate all answers directly to the job. Use standard English and avoid using slang. Many interviewers believe that the best predictor of future performance is past performance. Therefore, they will ask for details on your experience. Be prepared to give specific examples of past performance.

Stage 3: Questions from you. This is the time when questions from the health care interviewee are welcomed. You will have a few moments to sell yourself. Show that you are interested in the health care job by stressing your strengths and by mentioning qualities that might not have been discussed. Also, stress your willingness and eagerness to learn.

Be sure to ask questions about the job and the health care facility. Do not ask too many questions. Have a few thoughtfully prepared questions ready to refer to when asked. Employers are generally impressed when an applicant has good questions prepared in advance. Impress upon the interviewer that you would very much like to work for the health care facility.

Stage 4: Closing remarks. Watch for clues that indicate the interview has ended. Do not linger. Make a complimentary observation about the health care facility. "I am impressed with your health care facility's concern for its employees."

Often, you will not be offered a health care job immediately. If a decision cannot be made now, ask the employer what the next step in the process is. For example, some candidates might be called back for testing or a second interview. Ask when it would be convenient to call back about a hiring decision.

Shake the interviewer's hand and make your closing remark. Say, "I'm happy to have interviewed with you. Thank you for your time." This will leave a positive image.

DO'S AND DON'TS WHEN INTERVIEWING

Study the following list. Make a note of the items that you need to practice or review before your interview.

Do:

- Shake the interviewer's hand firmly when introduced.
- Be courteous. Say, "Good morning, Miss Kinoshita. I am John Stevens."
- Know the interviewer's name in advance; use the name in conversation with the interviewer.
- Remain standing until you are asked to sit down.
- Make yourself comfortable and maintain your poise.
- Present your resume to the interviewer. Leave it with him or her.
- Allow the interviewer to lead the interview.
- Look the interviewer in the eye.
- Answer all questions directly and truthfully.
- Use correct English. Avoid slang.
- Be agreeable at all times.
- Demonstrate your ability to take constructive criticism in a mature way.
- Show interest in the health care facility.
- Ask questions about the job opening and the health care facility.

- Make the interviewer aware of your goals and your sincerity about planning your health care career.
- Indicate a willingness to start at the bottom. Do not expect too much too soon.
- Express your appreciation for the interviewer's time.
- Take any examination requested.

Don't:

- Place your handbag, briefcase, or other articles on the interviewer's desk. (Keep them in your hands or place them on the floor beside you.)
- Slouch in your chair.
- Play with your tie, rings, bracelets, hair, etc.
- Chew gum.
- Smoke.
- Make excuses, be evasive, hedge on facts presented in your record.
- Answer a question before the question is completely asked.
- Interrupt the interviewer.
- Brag.
- Mumble.
- Make jokes or argue.
- Gossip or badmouth former employers.
- Ask too many questions.
- Beg for work.

A MODEL INTERVIEW

Carefully read the interview between Mr. Robert Allen, Human Resource Director, Danville Health Center, and job applicant Ms. Maria Lopez. This is a model case study. It is an ideal health care interview. Not all interviews are this smooth and perfect! The annotations highlight important benchmarks that occur in most interviews. Benchmarks are key points on which employers place special emphasis. When reading this model interview think about how you can incorporate these points in your health care interviews. You can observe and learn good interview skills by the way Maria conducts herself in the interview. She handles all aspects of the interview in a courteous manner. Maria takes an active role. She speaks with confidence and her confident attitude shows that she has done her homework. She describes her work skills well, reflects research of the health care facility, asks good questions, and is enthusiastic about the health care job. Maria is not passive. She speaks well and demonstrates she is a good prospect for employment. Maria's assertive role offers pointers that can be used in your interviews.

★ ★ **MEDICAL TRANSCRIPTIONIST** ★ ★
DIAGNOSTIC IMAGING

Excellent Career Opportunity with Danville Health Center in CA. Seeking qualified candidates to transcribe medical dictation such as X-ray reports, operative procedures, autopsies, pathology reports, medical histories, discharge summaries, and special clinical notes. Requirements: completion of a medical transcriber vocational training program or 6 mos. experience as a medical transcriber in hospital, medical institution, or professional medical transcription services may be substituted for the required vocational training. Some additional training available for qualified candidate. Several positions available, permanent and temporary. Vacation, sick leave, and holiday coverage. Send resume to Robert Allen, Human Resource Director, Danville Health Center, 1793 California Dr., Alamo, CA 94507-2407, or fax to (925) 555-8700.

Danville Health Center

An Equal Opportunity Employer

Figure 1-6-1 Danville Health Center Ad

Ms. Maria Lopez is seeking a medical record transcriptionist position that Danville Health Center has advertised in the newspaper ad, Figure 1-6-1. Maria has sent in her application, resume, and cover letter, and has been granted an interview. Maria walks into the office of Mr. Allen the interviewer.

Mr. Allen:
Hello, Maria, I'm Mr. Allen. Please be seated.

Get off to a good start.

Maria:
Thank you, Mr. Allen. I am happy to meet you.

Mr. Allen:
Welcome to Danville Health Center, Ms. Lopez. Did you have any trouble finding the Center?

Shows good preparation.

Maria:
No, last week I located your health care facility by driving here.

Mr. Allen:
That shows good planning on your part, Maria. According to your application and resume, you are interested in our medical record transcriptionist opening. Is that correct?

Maria:
Yes, Mr. Allen, I'd like to make a career in health care as a medical transcriptionist. I find such work challenging and exciting.

Mr. Allen:
Well, the job opening we have is in our medical records department. Your application indicates that you have extern training experience in medical transcription. Do you think you would like this type of work?

Maria:

Yes, I have always enjoyed secretarial work. Medical records are an important part of a person's well being, and it is important that these records be accurate. I would enjoy providing this service for Danville Health Center's staff and patients.

Mr. Allen:

Maria, since you have not had any employment in medical transcription, what qualifications do you think you have for this job?

Maria:

I am now working as an extern at Crestwood Hospital where I have received excellent transcription training. Many of the same secretarial skills I have developed at work, in high school, and at Bayview Medical/Dental Assisting College are used in transcribing these medical reports. Attention to detail, neatness, accuracy, and human relation skills are a few of my important responsibilities at Crestwood Hospital. I think that all of these responsibilities can be well applied to Danville's medical record transcription department.

This question invites you to talk about your work skills. Do you know all of yours?

Mr. Allen:

You're right. We need someone who has the skills and the responsibilities that you have described. You will soon graduate as a medical transcriptionist. How do you think your education has helped prepare you for this position?

Maria:

In high school I did well and enjoyed my keying, science, English, and drama classes. At Bayview Medical/Dental Assisting College I earned excellent grades in medical transcription, medical terminology, bookkeeping, and computer operation. My keying speed is 70 words per minute. In addition, my previous oral communication and drama classes helped me to gain confidence when speaking to others. I think I have developed skills from these courses that can be applied to the position of medical transcriptionist.

What school courses gave you useful skills?

Mr. Allen:

Yes, we need people with the right transcription and communication skills. If you were considered for this job opening, why would you want to work for Danville Health Center?

Maria:

Well, there is a branch of Danville Health Center located where I live, and I have come to depend on it for my health care needs. I find your branch health center convenient, cost effective, and efficient. In fact, many of my friends are with companies that subscribe to your health services for some of the same reasons.

I also did some research on large medical facilities. I discovered that Danville Health Center was one of the leaders in the field. It has an excellent reputation for quality service. I would very much like to work for a health center with this kind of reputation.

Note how Maria's good research shows and is appreciated.

Mr. Allen:

I see. It's nice to know you are familiar with Danville Health Center's services and its reputation. Is there any other reason you would like to work for our health facility?

Maria:

Yes, your center's annual brochure shows you are expanding statewide. This probably means that there will be opportunities for advancement.

Mr. Allen:

With the opening of the new Center—which has the job opening for which you applied—Danville Health Center plans to enlarge its network of health centers throughout the state. I think there will be many opportunities for advancement. We have just designed a new career management-training program which should accommodate our expansion. We will need more management people as our health care centers open.

Maria, for this job, we are looking for a person who can be on call for weekend work. Of course, when this is required, you would have an equal number of weekdays off. Would this be satisfactory for you?

Maria:

Show you have a flexible attitude.

Working weekends would be fine. At Crestwood Hospital I work every Saturday. It seems to me having weekdays off could be an advantage. Which days would I have off if I were to work weekends?

Mr. Allen:

You probably would have Mondays and Tuesdays off. The final decision will depend upon the needs of our medical transcription department.

Maria:

That would be fine with me.

Mr. Allen:

Will our new Danville Health Center be a convenient work location?

Maria:

The location of the new center would work out fine for me. I recently purchased a car and should have no problem.

Mr. Allen:

Maria, I see by your employment application you are presently working part-time for Hammond's Discount Bookstore. Have you enjoyed working for Hammond's?

Maria:

Yes, Mr. Allen, I have. For the past two years I have been employed as a part-time Hammond's employee while attending high school and Bayview Medical/Dental Assisting College. My part-time job has helped me pay for my education. Some of the skills that I have learned at Hammond's can be used in medical transcription work. Skills such as maintaining neat, complete, and accurate records are important in the book business. Good human relations are also necessary.

Mr. Allen:

Maria, do you have any questions you would like to ask?

Be prepared
to ask good
questions.

Maria:

Yes, can you give me more information about Danville's beginning employee training program and employee benefits package?

Mr. Allen:

All beginning employees start their training with a three-day welcome and orientation session. This covers our general operation and policies. After orientation, an employee is assigned to a department within the Center. There the starting employee receives on-the-job training. After this training is completed, the new employee is placed on probation for six months. Every two months during this probationary period, the department supervisor evaluates the employee. After successfully completing the probationary period, the new employee is classified as a "regular" employee and receives a raise in pay. Each regular employee is evaluated twice a year, generally every six months. After each successful evaluation, the employee earns a raise in pay. Our employee benefit package is standard for this industry. Danville gives holiday pay and two-week vacations after one year of service. We also give full medical and dental insurance coverage. Does that sufficiently explain what you wanted to know in these areas?

Maria:

Yes, thank you. That gives me some good information.

Mr. Allen:

We haven't discussed wages. What pay do you expect?

Maria does a
great job. She
does not ask for a
specific pay rate.

Maria:

Could you tell me what the pay range is for a beginning medical transcriptionist at Danville Health Center?

Mr. Allen:

Our pay range varies, depending on the department. For example, in our medical transcription department, the starting salary is $500.00 a week. After this, your pay is based on longevity and ability. Your supervisor will judge your ability level according to department standards. When your new employee orientation is scheduled, you will be given further details of this department wage and ability standard. How does that sound to you?

Maria:

That sounds very good.

Mr. Allen:

When could you start work if hired?

Maria:

I could start in two weeks, immediately after graduation from Bayview Medical/Dental Assisting College. When do you expect to complete interviewing for this position, Mr. Allen?

Mr. Allen:

I still have a few people left to interview, but I hope to be finished by next Tuesday.

> *Establish a follow-up phone call along with sending a post-interview letter.*

> *Sense when the interview is over and leave in a courteous and positive manner.*

Maria:

May I call you Wednesday morning? I am very interested in working for Danville Health Center. You have convinced me that Danville Health Center would make an excellent employer.

Mr. Allen:

Certainly. We would like you to follow up!

Maria:

Now that my interview is over, I am even more convinced that Danville is the health center for me. I really am impressed with its career possibilities. It was good talking with you. Thank you, Mr. Allen.

Mr. Allen:

You are welcome, Maria. Thank you for interviewing with Danville Health Center. Good-bye.

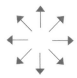

Activity Time!

Refer to Section 3—Activities.

CD-ROM

See Section 4 for directions.

ACTIVITY 10

HEALTH CARE CASE STUDY QUESTIONS

When you have finished reading the interview, remove Activity 10 in Section 3, and answer the case questions. By answering these questions, you will learn important interviewing skills. When you have completed this activity to your satisfaction, show it to your instructor for evaluation. Then place it in your employment portfolio for future health care interview preparation.

STEP 7
AFTER THE HEALTH CARE INTERVIEW

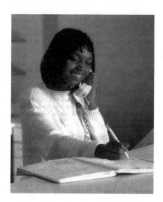

In this step you will find
- three ways to follow up on a job interview.
- a sample health care post-interview letter.
- an activity to construct a health care post-interview letter.
- how to evaluate a health care job offer.

WHY FOLLOW UP A HEALTH CARE INTERVIEW?

After all interviews for a health care position have been completed, there sometimes may be two or three equally qualified applicants for the one job opening. All of the applicants would probably make good employees, but only one may be selected. The selection will be difficult. However, one determining factor in making such a selection may be based on the applicant who exhibits the strongest desire or interest in the job. Therefore, the applicant who follows up on the interview may be the one selected for the job.

HOW DO YOU FOLLOW UP A HEALTH CARE JOB INTERVIEW?

You can follow up a health care job interview in three ways: You can make a return visit or a telephone call two or three days after the interview, or promptly send a post-interview letter. By making either a return visit, a phone call, or both, you can determine if a decision has been made and restate your interest in the position and in working for the health care facility. Here is a five-step follow-up plan when you call or revisit a health care facility.

1. **Reintroduce yourself and restate your interest in the job.**

   "Hello, Mrs. Vaughn. My name is Miguel Nieves. I interviewed with you last Wednesday for the job of Dental X-ray Technician. I wanted to thank you for discussing the position and let you know again that I would very much like to get the job."

2. **Add any additional thoughts you may not have covered when you interviewed.**

   "I did not mention in our interview my present plans for enrolling in a dental accounting class. Having some dental accounting background would be helpful when performing the job duties in a dental clinic."

3. Emphasize your strengths for the job.

"Mrs. Vaughn, the interview confirmed my belief that I have the skills required for the position of Dental X-ray Technician. My experience in dealing with people and my attention to detail are valuable skills that will be needed for this job. I also believe that the position of Dental X-ray Technician will be a challenging career opportunity."

4. Find out if a hiring decision has been made.

"Has a hiring decision been made for the position of Dental X-ray Technician?"

If a decision has been made and you did not get the job, ask the interviewer how you might have been a more competitive candidate. You could say, "I am sorry you don't feel I am the person for the job. At some future date I would like to interview again with your health care facility. Could you give me some suggestions for creating a better impression or for becoming a more qualified candidate?"

You may receive constructive criticism that will help you in future interviews. Make this a learning experience. Keep in mind, however, that health care facilities are not obligated to answer your question.

5. Thank the interviewer.

"Thank you for your time. I will wait for an answer."

Or, if you did not get the job, "Thank you for considering me for this position. I would appreciate your comments on my resume and interviewing skills."

The third method of following up the health care job interview is to write a post-interview letter. If you really want a particular health care job, write a letter immediately after the interview. Do not put this off! Pay as much attention to the quality and accuracy of this letter as your earlier correspondence. Proofread your letter before you mail it. If you have an error on this follow-up letter, you could lose your chance at a job you want. See Figure 1-7-1 for a sample health care post-interview letter. Read it carefully.

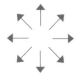

Activity Time!

Refer to Section 3—Activities.

CD-ROM

See Section 4 for directions.

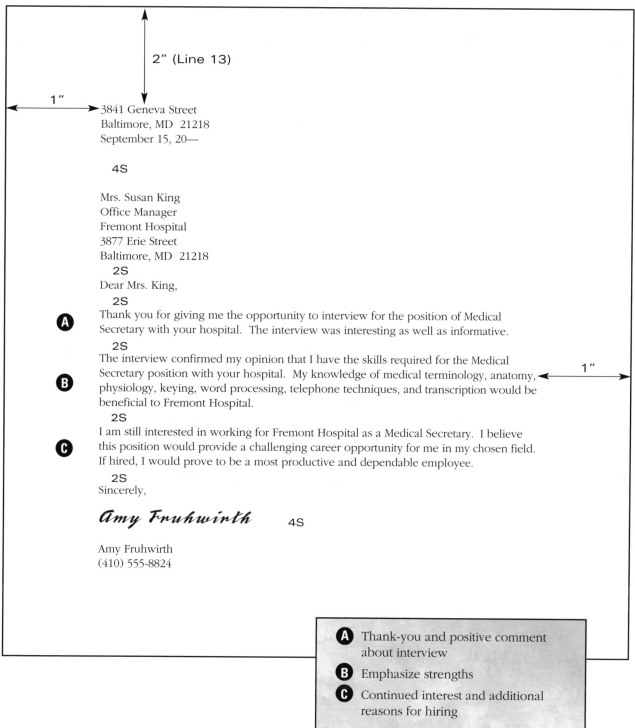

2" (Line 13)

1"

3841 Geneva Street
Baltimore, MD 21218
September 15, 20—

4S

Mrs. Susan King
Office Manager
Fremont Hospital
3877 Erie Street
Baltimore, MD 21218
2S
Dear Mrs. King,
2S

A Thank you for giving me the opportunity to interview for the position of Medical Secretary with your hospital. The interview was interesting as well as informative.
2S

B The interview confirmed my opinion that I have the skills required for the Medical Secretary position with your hospital. My knowledge of medical terminology, anatomy, physiology, keying, word processing, telephone techniques, and transcription would be beneficial to Fremont Hospital.
2S

1"

C I am still interested in working for Fremont Hospital as a Medical Secretary. I believe this position would provide a challenging career opportunity for me in my chosen field. If hired, I would prove to be a most productive and dependable employee.
2S
Sincerely,

Amy Fruhwirth   4S

Amy Fruhwirth
(410) 555-8824

A Thank-you and positive comment about interview

B Emphasize strengths

C Continued interest and additional reasons for hiring

Figure 1-7-1 Sample Post-Interview Letter

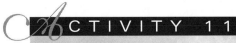

ACTIVITY 11

PREPARING A HEALTH CARE POST-INTERVIEW LETTER

Based on the information in the following scenario, remove Activity 11 in Section 3, and draft a post-interview letter. Refer to the sample letter, Figure 1-7-1, to complete this health care post-interview letter. After you have drafted the letter, show it to your instructor for evaluation. Key and save your letter on the same disk that has your resume and other material from this manual. Print your final letter on white 8 1/2" x 11" paper. Place your printed post-interview letter and computer disk in your employment portfolio for future reference.

Scenario for Activity 11

You have interviewed for the health care job of (insert your job choice). The job pays well. The working conditions and hours meet your needs and you are a good prospect for this position. Mr. David Souza, the personnel manager, has told you that he has other applicants to interview. You have decided to follow up with a post-interview letter to Mr. David Souza, the Personnel Manager. His employment address is St. Louis Medical/Dental Clinic, 200 Washington Avenue, St. Louis, MO 63103. You may use a health care facility of your choice if you prefer. Your local newspaper's employment section will list other health care facilities and positions for this post-interview letter.

EVALUATING A HEALTH CARE JOB OFFER

Congratulations! Your hard work has paid off. You are offered the health care job. Now you will have to decide whether or not to accept it. This decision should be an easy one to make if you have gathered the necessary information about the health care facility and the position, and if you have evaluated the job's advantages and disadvantages.

The information you have gathered, along with the following questions, will help you make the right decision.

1. Does this health care position provide the kind of work that will be satisfying day after day?
2. Can you live on the wages being offered?
3. How are wage increases earned?
4. Does the health care facility offer satisfactory job security? Job security is how the health care facility deals with lay-offs and other unemployment issues.
5. Is the health care facility's benefit package satisfactory?
6. Is your supervisor the kind of person for whom you could easily work?
7. Are the co-workers the kind of people with whom you could easily work?
8. Is the health care facility location convenient?
9. Does this health care job offer opportunities for training, education, and advancement?

SECTION

2

Leaving a Health Care Job... Gracefully

INTRODUCTION

The three steps in Section 2 contain valuable advice and insight concerning how to leave a job in health care gracefully and with excellent references. There is far more to leaving a job than saying, "I quit." This section includes procedures and activities that will end your health care job on a positive note.

The three steps in Section 2, Leaving a Health Care Job...Gracefully, follow, along with a summary of what each step includes.

Step 1: Questions to Consider Before Leaving a Health Care Job

This step presents important questions you should ask yourself before leaving a health care job.

Step 2: The Best Way to Leave a Health Care Job

This step explains the positive way to leave a health care job. You will learn what to say to your employer and how to write a resignation letter.

Step 3: Health Care Reference Letter

This step shows you how to obtain a reference letter which can be used to obtain future jobs.

Special Circumstances: When You Must Leave a Health Care Job

This section ends by outlining positive procedures for handling serious employment problems. If you are laid off, downsized, or fired, this information is essential.

STEP 1
QUESTIONS TO CONSIDER BEFORE LEAVING A HEALTH CARE JOB

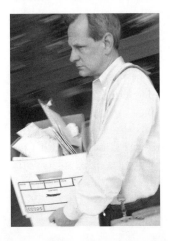

In this step you will find

- information on when to leave a health care job.
- questions to consider before leaving a health care job.
- how to compare advantages and disadvantages of a health care job.
- a quiz to help you decide if you should leave a health care job.
- a health care case study activity.

WHY DOES SOMEONE LEAVE A HEALTH CARE JOB?

Each month more than a million Americans make a job change. People have many reasons for deciding to leave a health care employer. These include

- finding another health care job that shows more promise or pays better.
- no longer feeling satisfaction with the health care work.
- having been passed over for promotion.
- wishing to make a health care career change.
- having the job affect health.
- having important responsibilities taken away.
- experiencing organizational downsizing.
- being in a position where retirement is an option.

FIVE QUESTIONS TO CONSIDER BEFORE LEAVING A HEALTH CARE JOB

Choosing to leave a health care job can be a very emotional, stressful decision. It can cause insecurity and a loss of career movement. You should understand why you want to leave. Ask yourself if you have done everything you can to improve or to make the most of your current health care situation. Consider the following:

1. If your health care job is not satisfying or challenging, have you spoken to your boss about making your job more satisfying? Have you looked into changing jobs within your health care facility? Have you applied for additional training, education, or special health care programs? Are there promotional opportunities?

2. What is the financial impact of your decision? At this time, can you afford to leave this health care job? Can you obtain a comparable health care job that will provide equal or higher pay and benefits? What benefits will you lose (medical, dental, etc.) and can you afford to lose them? Not all financial decisions are short term. You should also consider what impact leaving your health care employment would have on long-term benefits such as retirement and employee profit sharing plans.

3. Have you done everything possible to resolve any personality conflicts with your supervisor or fellow health care employees? Have you discussed these conflicts with your supervisor or the person with whom you are having the conflict? Is it possible that this person will eventually be transferred out of your work area?

4. What is it about your environment that you don't like? Examples of work conditions include having a comfortable and well-equipped workspace where health and safety standards are met. Have you discussed ways to improve the environment with your supervisor? If they can't be improved, is it possible to transfer to another workstation within your health care facility?

5. What impact will leaving your health care job have on your career plans? If you are considering employment with another health care facility, what do you know about the facility's financial condition, goals and objectives, management philosophy, and competition? Have you compared these features with your present health care facility?

To decide when it is time to leave, it may help to make a list of the advantages and disadvantages of your current health care employment situation. Or you can take the quiz in Figure 2-1-1 to help you think through your decision.

Trust Your Instincts

If you go through the steps suggested here, you will know when it is right to leave a health care job. Respect your inner feelings with regard to your employment. Since your health care job represents a large portion of your daily life, it is important to feel good about what you are doing.

Regardless of your reason, never let leaving become a negative, stressful experience. If a paycheck is necessary, make sure you have another job, or at least the promise of one, before leaving. You can use the techniques in Section 1 of this manual to find a health care job whether you are currently employed or not.

Is It Time for a Health Care Job Change?
Ten Questions to Help You Decide

Whenever you are wondering if it is time to change a health care job, take the following ten-question quiz. Check (✔) a yes or no box for each question. When you have completed the quiz, add your yes and no answers. If you have answered **more** questions *yes* than *no,* you may be ready for a health care employment change.

Yes No

☐ ☐ 1. Does your health care manager ignore your suggestions?

☐ ☐ 2. Have you been passed over consistently for a promotion?

☐ ☐ 3. Do you feel underpaid for work you perform?

☐ ☐ 4. Is your health care employment harming your physical or emotional health?

☐ ☐ 5. Do you find yourself constantly watching the clock at work?

☐ ☐ 6. Are promises made to you by your health care employer but not kept?

☐ ☐ 7. Have you received poor performance evaluations?

☐ ☐ 8. Would your co-workers say you are a difficult person with whom to work?

☐ ☐ 9. Do you feel unrecognized for your good work?

☐ ☐ 10. Do you have more bad workdays than good?

Figure 2-1-1 Ten-Question Quiz

Activity Time!
Refer to Section 3—Activities.

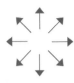

CD-ROM
See Section 4 for directions.

ACTIVITY 12

HEALTH CARE CASE STUDY—DECISION TIME

Carefully read the case study about Peter Chang. Peter needs your help to decide what to do about his health care job. Remove the activity worksheet provided, and create a list showing the advantages and disadvantages of Peter remaining in his current employment. Decide for yourself what his decision should be. If you decide Peter should remain, tell what he could do to improve his health care job situation. Be sure to review the *Five Questions To Consider Before Leaving A Health Care Job* and the *Five Fast Ways You Can Improve Health Care Employment Satisfaction,* found in this step, to suggest what Peter should do. When you have completed this activity to your satisfaction, show it to your instructor for evaluation and class discussion. Now you know the questions to ask yourself, and a process to follow, before leaving a health care job. Refer to the questions in this step when deciding if you should keep or leave a health care job in the future.

FIVE FAST WAYS YOU CAN IMPROVE HEALTH CARE EMPLOYMENT SATISFACTION

1. Maintain a good attitude.

2. Keep a good balance between your health care employment and personal life.

3. Learn new skills to increase your value to your health care facility.

4. Improve any human relation problems you have at your health care facility.

5. Redesign your work.

STEP 2
THE BEST WAY TO LEAVE A HEALTH CARE JOB

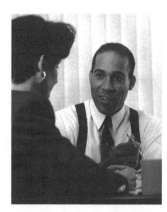

In this step you will find

- positive ways to leave a health care job.
- what to tell your health care employer.
- what to tell your co-workers.
- a sample health care resignation letter.
- a health care resignation letter activity.
- a health care exit conversation activity.

POSITIVE WAYS TO LEAVE A HEALTH CARE JOB

Your employer expects you to know how to end your health care employment in a positive, mature way. Do not feel you are doing the wrong thing by leaving. According to U.S. government statistics, the average person will have six or seven different jobs during a lifetime. Since your first job probably will not be your last, it is important to know how to leave a health care job in a positive way.

Leaving a health care job in a businesslike manner protects your reputation and may help you obtain a favorable reference. Keep the door open for future business dealings you may have with your former health care employer. Perhaps one day you may even want to rejoin your old organization or work with a former supervisor or co-worker at another health care facility. Following are points you will want to use when leaving a health care job.

Follow Organization Policy

Usually two weeks notice is expected, although some health care employers may require more or less time in order to hire and train your replacement. Your health care employer will appreciate an offer to help train your replacement and will most likely remember your spirit of cooperation. This could definitely influence the type of reference you receive.

Write a Health Care Resignation Letter

This letter informs your health care employer and/or supervisor of your decision to leave. Present this letter to your supervisor before telling your co-workers and friends about your leaving. You do not want your employer to find out that you are leaving from another employee. A well-written health care resignation letter could lead to a good recommendation. Be sure to include the following required elements.

- the date you wish to leave your health care facility
- your reasons for leaving a health care job (keep them positive)
- your thanks for the skills you have learned
- your appreciation of the people with whom you have worked

Figure 2-2-1 provides a good example of a well-written resignation letter. Study it carefully.

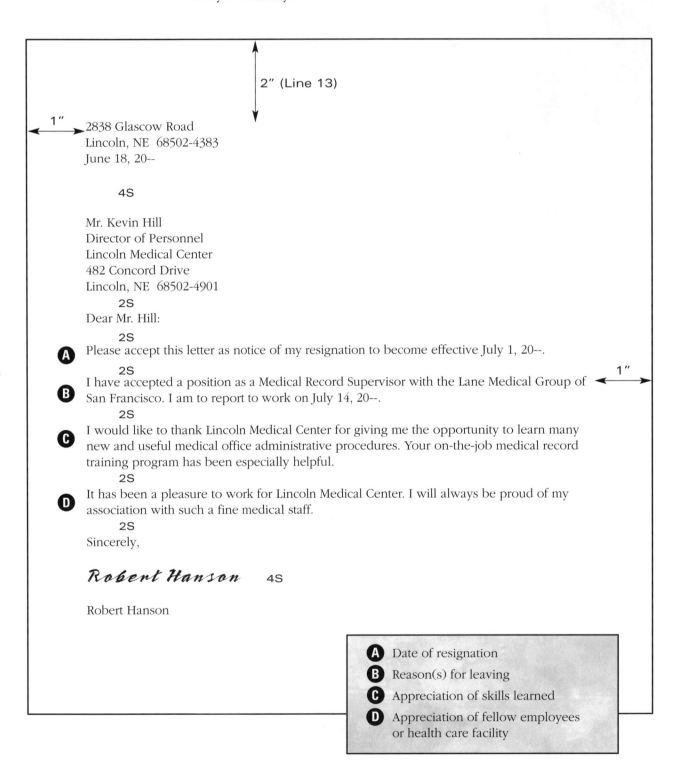

2″ (Line 13)

1″

2838 Glascow Road
Lincoln, NE 68502-4383
June 18, 20--

4S

Mr. Kevin Hill
Director of Personnel
Lincoln Medical Center
482 Concord Drive
Lincoln, NE 68502-4901
2S
Dear Mr. Hill:
2S

A Please accept this letter as notice of my resignation to become effective July 1, 20--.
2S

B I have accepted a position as a Medical Record Supervisor with the Lane Medical Group of San Francisco. I am to report to work on July 14, 20--.
2S

C I would like to thank Lincoln Medical Center for giving me the opportunity to learn many new and useful medical office administrative procedures. Your on-the-job medical record training program has been especially helpful.
2S

D It has been a pleasure to work for Lincoln Medical Center. I will always be proud of my association with such a fine medical staff.
2S
Sincerely,

Robert Hanson   4S

Robert Hanson

1″

A Date of resignation
B Reason(s) for leaving
C Appreciation of skills learned
D Appreciation of fellow employees or health care facility

Figure 2-2-1 Sample Resignation Letter

THE EXIT INTERVIEW: WHAT TO TELL YOUR HEALTH CARE EMPLOYER

Many health care facilities have formal exit interviews for employees who have resigned. These interviews may be completed with your health care supervisor or with someone from the human relations department.

Job Skills I Have Learned

_____

_____

_____

_____

Work Habits I Have Improved

_____

_____

_____

_____

When you hand in your resignation letter, your supervisor will expect you to tell why you are leaving. Prepare yourself. Before you have your exit interview make a list of some positive things you have learned from your health care job. Think hard! Your experience may have taught you job skills such as business operation software, medical office bookkeeping, communication skills, laboratory techniques, safety precautions, etc. Your job may have also improved such work habits as communicating well with other people, performing work with minimal instructions, following orders, being responsible, being dependable, dealing with patients in a positive way, and being able to work under pressure.

A MODEL HEALTH CARE EXIT CONVERSATION

The following conversation is a good example of how to inform your health care employer that you are leaving your job. Note that Paul's exit conversation is short and to the point. He is polite and leaves a positive impression.

"Ms. Choi, it is necessary for me to give you and Seagate Medical Center notice that I am leaving. (Hands letter of resignation to Ms. Choi.) I have enjoyed working with the many great people that make up this health care facility. I have accepted a position with Kirkland Medical Group as Medical Records Supervisor. By making this change, I will be able to develop and improve my medical record knowledge and management skills.

I want to thank you for the excellent medical office administration experience I have received working for Seagate Medical Center. I have learned the importance of sound health care organizational strategies and effective leadership skills.

Would you like me to train my replacement?"

WHAT TO TELL YOUR CO-WORKERS

After you have told your health care employer that you leaving and submitted your resignation letter, you should also tell your fellow employees. Keep your remarks short and reasons for leaving positive. Make sure your reasons for leaving are the same positive ones you expressed to management. Tell your fellow employees that it was great working with them and you will miss them. Whatever you do, don't brag about any greater benefits of your new job. Your co-workers may become jealous. Save those comments for your family and close friends not associated with your health care facility. Out of fairness to your health care organization and co-workers, do not mention any negative conditions about the job you are leaving. This will reflect poorly on you. Your fellow workers will not appreciate negative remarks about their health care employer.

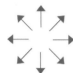

Activity Time!
Refer to Section 3—Activities.

CD-ROM
See Section 4 for directions.

ACTIVITY 13

WRITE A HEALTH CARE RESIGNATION LETTER

Carefully read the sample health care resignation letter in this step. Remember a time that you left a job or assume that you are resigning from a health care position where you have been successful and learned a great deal. Using the sample health care resignation letter as a guide, write your own health care resignation letter. Remove the Activity 13 worksheet provided in Section 3. After you have drafted your letter, show it to your instructor for evaluation. Key your final health care resignation letter and save the file to the same computer disk as your resume and other documents from this manual. Place a printed copy of your health care resignation letter and the computer disk in your employment portfolio. Remember that when you leave a health care job, you should also update your resume with new skills that you have achieved.

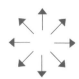

Activity Time!

Refer to Section 3—Activities.

CD-ROM

See Section 4 for directions.

ACTIVITY 14
EXIT CONVERSATION

Using Paul's model health care exit conversation as a guide, write your own exit conversation. Address your conversation to either a present or a past employer. If you have never held a job, select any health care employer. Remember to be discreet and keep your exit conversation short and to the point. Remove the paper provided for Activity 14 in Section 3, and write your exit conversation. After you have written your health care exit conversation, show it to your instructor for evaluation. Place your completed exit conversation in your employment portfolio for future reference.

STEP 3
HEALTH CARE REFERENCE LETTER

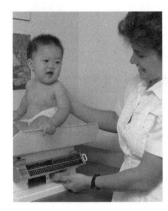

In this step you will find

- what a health care reference letter is.
- how to get a health care reference letter.
- a sample health care reference letter.
- a health care reference letter activity.

WHAT IS A HEALTH CARE REFERENCE LETTER?

A health care reference letter contains statements about your character, abilities, skills, and attitudes. It can be a valuable tool for future health care job interviews. You will use this health care reference letter when applying for future health care jobs by attaching a copy to your employment application, resume, or post-interview letter. You may also want to present your reference letter during your health care job interviews. Always keep your original letter. Distribute copies only.

HOW TO GET A HEALTH CARE REFERENCE LETTER

Before leaving a health care job, ask your employer or supervisor for a reference letter or letter of recommendation. Sometimes employers are very busy and they will ask you to prepare your own reference letter, which they may edit and then sign. Usually they will suggest some of the points they would include in the letter. If they don't, ask them if there is anything they would like to say about you in the letter. Do not pass up this opportunity to present the very best side of yourself.

An example of a good health care reference letter is shown in Figure 2-3-1. Notice that the letter is specific about Robert's contributions to the health care facility and mentions positive personality traits.

You should try to have a reference letter in your portfolio from each of your health care employers. Reference letters may not, however, be enough for prospective health care employers. You should also have health care references with whom a prospective employer can make personal contact. Ask your health care employer to include in his or her reference letter an invitation to readers to call for more details.

Activity Time!
Refer to Section 3—Activities.

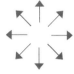

CD-ROM
See Section 4 for directions.

1 1/2"

LINCOLN
✚ MEDICAL CENTER
482 Concord Drive / Lincoln, NE 68502-4901
(402) 555-2888

4S

1"

July 9, 20--

4S

To Whom It May Concern,

2S

A Robert Hanson was a Medical Record employee with Lincoln Medical Center for the past
three years. As a Medical Record employee, he displayed many excellent leadership and
productivity skills. His timely suggestions for reducing telemarketing costs led to increased
profits for our Medical Center.

1"

2S

B Besides being very helpful, Robert is responsible and gets along well with his co-workers.
I would highly recommend Robert Hanson as an excellent employee.

2S

C Please call me at (402) 555-0123 if you would like to speak to me directly about Robert's
contributions to the company.

2S

Sincerely,

Kevin Hill 4S

Kevin Hill
Director of Personnel

A Abilities, skills, and
accomplishments

B Attitude and character

C Invitation to reader to call for more
details

Figure 2-3-1 Sample Reference Letter

ACTIVITY 15

CONSTRUCT A HEALTH CARE REFERENCE LETTER

Use your present job or think about a job you've had (it may have been a paid job with a company, work done for a health care facility, or volunteer work). Using the sample health care reference letter as a guide, remove Activity 15 in Section 3, and write yourself a health care reference letter. (If you've never had a job with a company or health care facility, write a reference letter for yourself to be signed by an instructor or supervisor who could write you a letter of reference based on your participation in a classroom, as a volunteer, or other group association.)

When you have finished writing your health care reference letter, show it to your instructor for evaluation. Then key your completed health care reference letter on a good grade of white 8 1/2" x 11" paper. You have now learned how to construct a health care reference letter. Place the completed reference letter in your employment portfolio along with your computer disk.

SPECIAL CIRCUMSTANCES: WHEN YOU MUST LEAVE A HEALTH CARE JOB

Unless you are very lucky, you probably won't always be able to leave a health care job on your own schedule. You may be laid off, downsized, or fired. This last section of *How to Get a Job in Health Care* includes some suggestions for making the best of these difficult situations.

WHAT TO DO IF YOU ARE LAID OFF OR DOWNSIZED

Laid off means to be put out of work due to no fault of your own. Frequently a general layoff is temporary. If you are laid off, you have two choices: wait until your health care job reopens or find another health care job. Before you decide to wait until your health care job reopens, find out what your chances are for being rehired. If you decide to wait until you are called back, plan your time and financial resources carefully.

If you decide to find another health care job, ask your employer for a reference letter. This letter could help you during your next health care job interview. Some health care facilities have policies about not giving out references (to avoid lawsuits). You should have several sources as references.

Being downsized means that the health care facility has decided to reduce its labor force. If you are a victim of downsizing, you are unemployed due to no fault of your own. You need to immediately look for another health care job.

WHAT TO DO IF YOU ARE FIRED

Being fired is a serious matter. As a reaction to this unpleasant experience, your self-esteem and confidence may suffer, but it is not the end of your working career. Many people have been fired from health care jobs. There are many reasons a person may be fired. Some common reasons are poor performance, poor work habits, negative attitude, personality conflicts, falsifying health care facility documents, and violations of the health care facility policy.

If you are fired, it is important to learn something from the experience and to take responsibility for it. Ask your health care employer to explain the reasons for firing you. Carefully examine these reasons and don't make excuses. Ask yourself the following:

- If poor performance was a problem, do I need more medical training?
- Did I not fully understand the health care job requirements when I was hired?
- Did the health care job requirements change?
- Did personality problems affect my work?
- Do I need to change certain work habits and attitudes in order to meet the expectations of another health care employer?

You should answer these questions for yourself before you begin your next health care job search.

What Do You Tell Prospective Employers?

Should you mention being fired on a health care employment application or during future health care interviews? You, of course, are the only one who can answer this question. Revealing being fired to possible health care employers might not be in your best interests. Many individuals who have been fired simply say that they are making a change for career opportunity or seeking employment in another type of health care facility. In most cases, this type of positive comment satisfies the question, "Why did you leave your last health care job?" If a person is not truthful, and they get hired, they could subsequently be fired for providing false information.

A health care employer may find out you were fired in the course of checking your references. If this embarrassing question arises, handle it calmly. What you say and the manner in which you say it are extremely important. Be honest about your reason for leaving and acknowledge your mistakes. Show ownership and responsibility for what happened. Do not blame your health care employer.

Explain what you learned from the experience. You might add that, because of what you learned from being fired, you are now prepared to be a better employee. Your next health care employer may be more willing to give you a chance if you are sincerely trying to improve your job performance.

Assume that you have been fired from your health care job. Although you regret the decision, you agree with your health care employer's reasoning. From the information you have learned, answer the questions presented here.

1. What actions would you take if you were fired?

_____

_____

_____

_____

2. What questions should you answer for yourself before you look for another health care job?

_____

_____

_____

_____

3. What would you say to the health care employer who fired you?

_____

_____

_____

_____

4. If fired from a health care job, what reasons for leaving would you place on an employment application?

_____

_____

_____

_____

5. What would you say to a health care facility interviewer who discovered that you were fired from your last health care job and asked for an explanation?

_____

_____

_____

_____

Using the Seven-Step Process to Get Another Health Care Job

Whenever you leave a job, you should follow the seven-step process found in Section 1 of _How to Get a Job in Health Care_ to find a new one. Begin by updating your resume. Even if you left your health care job under unpleasant circumstances, you have probably sharpened or acquired new medical related skills as well as experience. Identify and pursue as many health care job leads as you can. You may want to practice interview situations to discuss why you left your last health care job. Whatever you do, don't give up. There is a good health care job that is right for you. Your first task is to find it.

SECTION

3

Getting and Leaving a Job in Health Care— Activities

INTRODUCTION

The activities in Section 3 of *How to Get a Job in Health Care* are provided to assist you in completing the steps in Sections 1 and 2. These activities provide valuable documents for employment in the health care industry. Be sure to establish an employment portfolio, to use as a file, to keep your completed activities. Place the completed activities in your employment portfolio to reference when you are securing or leaving future health care positions.

The following activities are for the seven steps in Section 1: Getting a Job in Health Care, and the three steps in Section 2: Leaving a Health Care Job...Gracefully.

Section 1: Getting a Job in Health Care

Step Number	Activity Number	Activity Title
1	1	Checklist of Employment Power Words and Phrases
1	2	Writing Health Care Job Objectives
1	3	Constructing a Health Care Resume
1	4	Constructing a Health Care Reference List
2	5	Writing a Health Care Cover Letter
3	6	Completing a Health Care Employment Application
4	7	Finding Health Care Job Leads
4	8	Researching a Health Care Facility
5	9	Answering Interview Questions
6	10	Health Care Case Study Questions
7	11	Preparing a Health Care Post-Interview Letter

Section 2: Leaving a Health Care Job...Gracefully

Step Number	Activity Number	Activity Title
1	12	Health Care Case Study—Decision Time
2	13	Writing a Health Care Resignation Letter
2	14	Health Care Exit Conversation
3	15	Constructing a Health Care Reference Letter

Name _____ Date _____

SECTION 1 STEP 1
HEALTH CARE RESUME (PERSONAL DATASHEET)

𝒜CTIVITY 1
CHECKLIST OF EMPLOYMENT POWER WORDS AND PHRASES

Directions: The following Employment Power Words Checklist contains many assertive and action words and phrases that health care employers want to hear. Use these words and phrases to help write an effective resume, cover letter, employment application, post-interview letter, reference letter, and resignation letter. These power words can also be very helpful to project a positive, confident image at your interview. When you have completed this to your satisfaction, show it to your instructor for evaluation. With this activity you establish your employment portfolio. It can be as simple as a file folder. It will contain this completed activity and other important documents, such as your resume and reference list, that you complete in this manual. They all can be used for future reference in getting and leaving a job in health care.

EMPLOYMENT POWER WORDS AND PHRASES CHECKLIST

Place a check mark (✓) next to the power words and phrases that you feel describe you best.

I am able to:

_____ communicate effectively	_____ pay attention to detail
_____ pre-plan	_____ set priorities
_____ analyze materials	_____ meet deadlines
_____ budget time and resources	_____ notice important details
_____ follow instructions	_____ organize my work
_____ motivate others	_____ persistently learn
_____ make good decisions	_____ handle public relations
_____ be dedicated	_____ be dependable
_____ keep up with current changes	_____ take responsibility
_____ easily work with others	_____ promote projects
_____ be enthusiastic	_____ research materials
_____ estimate accurately	_____ be a problem solver
_____ be thorough	_____ teach others
_____ be an excellent team member	_____ expedite work
_____ work easily with a computer	_____ remember details
_____ manage others	_____ be a leader
_____ follow health office procedures	_____ read and understand data quickly
_____ perform well under pressure	_____ work easily with instruments
_____ be goal-oriented	_____ work easily with machines
_____ be a self-starter	_____ work independently

List other traits you have that are beneficial in a health care position.

_____

_____

_____

_____

_____

Look at the power words and phrases you have checked and listed. Select five that best describe you, and write them here.

1. _____

2. _____

3. _____

4. _____

5. _____

Using these five power words and phrases, write a paragraph telling a prospective employer why you should be hired.

_____

_____

_____

_____

_____

_____

_____

_____

_____

_____

_____

_____

_____

_____

_____

_____

_____

_____

Name _____ Date _____

SECTION 1 STEP 1
HEALTH CARE RESUME (PERSONAL DATASHEET)

ACTIVITY 2
WRITING HEALTH CARE JOB OBJECTIVES

Directions: Write a job objective for each of the medical-related employment ads presented here. Then complete this activity by writing your own job objective for the health care job you would like. Remember, a job objective can be for a specific health care job title, type of health care work, or a medical-related career goal.

Your health care job objectives should be clear and concisely written. Use the example of health care job objectives in Section 1, Step 1 as a guide. When you have written your health care job objectives to your satisfaction, show them to your instructor for evaluation. Place your completed health care job objective worksheet in your employment portfolio for future reference.

X-RAY TECHNICIAN

Competitive salary plus excellent benefit package; HIRE-ON BONUS & MOVING ALLOWANCE AVAILABLE. Immediate opening for a full-time technician to perform X-ray work. Acute care facility in beautiful Mendocino Country in the heart of the redwoods region with ocean and lake access. Must be a dependable team player with current registration as an X-ray technician. X-ray exp. preferred. Call for more information, send/fax/e-mail resume, or apply in person. EOE

UNITED MEDICAL CENTER
275 Morgan Drive
Ukiah, CA 95482
(707) 555-8484 or Fax (707) 555-2323
Attn: Human Resources
flowermr@nvbo.org

Health care position applying for: _____

_____

Health care job objective: _____

_____

_____

_____

❀ ❀ **MEDICAL** ❀ ❀

Receptionist/Scheduler needed to work in our out-patient and hospital based radiology offices in Alamo and Danville. We offer competitive salary and benefits. Medical experience required. Please fax resume to (925) 555-2424 or e-mail to hbana@bnni.net

Health care position applying for: _____

_____

Health care job objective: _____

_____
_____
_____

**MEDICAL
TRANSCRIPTIONIST**

Radiology bkgd. P/T to F/T with variable hours. Fax resume to (415) 555-0852. Mercy Hospital

Health care position applying for: _____

_____

Health care job objective: _____

_____
_____
_____

Now think of the health care job you want and complete the following:

The health care position I am applying for: _____

_____

My health care job objective: _____

_____
_____
_____

Name _____ Date _____

SECTION 1 STEP **1**
HEALTH CARE RESUME (PERSONAL DATASHEET)

ACTIVITY 3
CONSTRUCTING A HEALTH CARE RESUME—
STANDARD RESUME (PRACTICE SHEET)

Directions: Gather information about your education and work experience. Complete this outline by writing your resume information on the lines below. When you have completed this outline to your satisfaction, show it to your instructor for evaluation. Next, using this completed outline as a guide, key your resume. Use the sample standard resume in Figure 1-1-2 in Section 1, Step 1, as a reference and spacing guide. Save your resume to a disk for easy updating. Keep it updated as you gain experience and education. Place your completed resume and computer disk with the saved resume file in your employment portfolio.

PERSONAL INFORMATION

_____
(Name)
_____
(Address)
_____
(City, State, Zip code)
(____)_____
(Telephone and Fax Number, E-mail Address)

JOB OBJECTIVE

_____

_____

_____

EDUCATION
(List most recent school first.)

_____
(Month, Year to Month, Year)

_____
(School Name)
_____
(Address)
_____
(City, State, Zip Code)
_____
(Program)
_____
(Degree)
Courses: _____

_____

_____

_____

_____
(Month, Year to Month, Year)

_____
(School Name)

_____
(Address)

_____
(City, State, Zip Code)

_____
(Program)

_____
(Degree)

Courses: _____

_____

_____

_____

WORK EXPERIENCE
(List most recent work experience first.)

_____
(Month, Year to Month, Year)

_____
(Company/Health Care Facility Name)

_____
(Address)

_____
(City, State, Zip Code)

_____
(Job Title)

Responsibilities: _____

_____

_____
(Month, Year to Month, Year)

_____
(Company/Health Care Facility Name)

_____
(Address)

_____
(City, State, Zip Code)

_____
(Job Title)

Responsibilities: _____

_____

MEMBERSHIPS

_____

_____

HONORS

_____

_____

SPECIAL SKILLS

_____

_____

REFERENCES

References available on request.

Name _____ Date _____

SECTION 1 STEP **1**
HEALTH CARE RESUME (PERSONAL DATASHEET)

CTIVITY 3
CONSTRUCTING A HEALTH CARE RESUME— CHRONOLOGICAL RESUME (PRACTICE SHEET)

Directions: Gather information about your education and work experience. Complete this outline by writing your resume information on the lines below. When you have completed this outline to your satisfaction, show it to your instructor for evaluation. Next, using this completed outline as a guide, key your resume. Use the sample chronological resume in Figure 1-1-3 in Section 1, Step 1, as a reference and spacing guide. Save your resume to a disk for easy updating. Keep it updated as you gain experience and education. Place your completed resume and computer disk with the saved resume file in your employment portfolio.

_____
(Name)
_____
(Address)
_____
(City, State, Zip Code)
( ) _____
(Telephone Number)

JOB OBJECTIVE

_____
_____
_____
_____

QUALIFICATIONS

_____
_____
_____
_____
_____
_____

EMPLOYERS

_____
(Month, Year to Month, Year)

_____
(Company Name)

_____
(City, State)

_____
(Job Title)

_____
(Month, Year to Month, Year)

_____
(Company Name)

_____
(City, State)

_____
(Job Title)

_____
(Month, Year to Month, Year)

_____
(Company Name)

_____
(City, State)

_____
(Job Title)

REFERENCES

References available on request.

Name _____ Date _____

SECTION 1 STEP 1
HEALTH CARE RESUME (PERSONAL DATASHEET)

ACTIVITY 3
CONSTRUCTING A HEALTH CARE RESUME—
FUNCTIONAL RESUME (PRACTICE SHEET)

Directions: Gather information about your education and work experience. Complete this outline by writing your resume information on the lines below. When you have completed this outline to your satisfaction, show it to your instructor for evaluation. Next, using this completed outline as a guide, key your resume. Use the sample functional resume in Figure 1-1-4 in Section 1, Step 1, as a reference and spacing guide. Save your resume to a disk for easy updating. Keep it updated as you gain experience and education. Place your completed resume and computer disk with the saved resume file in your employment portfolio.

_____
(Name)
_____
(Address)
_____
(City, State, Zip Code)
(   ) _____
(Telephone Number)

JOB OBJECTIVE _____
_____
_____
_____

EXPERIENCE

_____
(Job Title)

_____
(Company/Health Care Facility/Organization Name)
_____
(City, State)
_____
(Skills in paragraph form)
_____
_____
_____
_____
_____

_____   _____
(Job Title)   (Company/Health Care Facility/Organization Name)

                            _____
                            (City, State)

                            _____
                            (Skills in paragraph form)

                            _____

                            _____

                            _____

                            _____

                            _____

                            _____

_____   _____
(Job Title)   (Company/Health Care Facility/Organization Name)

                            _____
                            (City, State)

                            _____
                            (Skills in paragraph form)

                            _____

                            _____

                            _____

                            _____

                            _____

                            _____

EDUCATION

                            _____
                            (School Name)

                            _____
                            (City, State)

                            _____
                            (Degree and Major)

                            _____
                            (School Name)

                            _____
                            (City, State)

                            _____
                            (Degree and Major)

                            _____
                            (School Name)

                            _____
                            (City, State)

                            _____
                            (Degree and Major)

REFERENCES

References available on request.

Name _____ Date _____

STEP 1

HEALTH CARE RESUME (PERSONAL DATASHEET)

ACTIVITY 3

CONSTRUCTING A HEALTH CARE RESUME—
COMBINATION RESUME (PRACTICE SHEET)

Directions: Gather information about your education and work experience. Complete this outline by writing your resume information on the lines below. When you have completed this outline to your satisfaction, show it to your instructor for evaluation. Next, using this completed outline as a guide, key your resume. Use the sample combination resume in Figure 1-1-5 in Section 1, Step 1, as a reference and spacing guide. Save your resume to a disk for easy updating. Keep it updated as you gain experience and education. Place your completed resume and computer disk with the saved resume file in your employment portfolio.

_____
(Name)
_____
(Address)
_____
(City, State, Zip Code)
(   )
_____
(Telephone Number)

WORK EXPERIENCE

_____   _____
(Job Title)   (Company/Health Care Facility/Organization Name, City, State)
_____   _____
(Month, Year to Month, Year)   (Duties)
                                _____
                                _____
                                _____

_____   _____
(Job Title)   (Company/Health Care Facility/Organization Name, City, State)
_____   _____
(Month, Year to Month, Year)   (Duties)
                                _____
                                _____

EDUCATION

_____
(Degree/Certificate, School, City, State)
_____

Graduated _____, 20_____. _____
         (month)

_____

_____

_____

_____

_____

_____

_____

_____

(Degree/Certificate, School, City, State)

_____

Graduated _____, 20_____. _____
         (month)

_____

_____

_____

_____

_____

_____

_____

REFERENCES   References available on request.

Name _____ Date _____

SECTION 1 STEP 1
HEALTH CARE RESUME (PERSONAL DATASHEET)

ACTIVITY 4
CONSTRUCTING A HEALTH CARE REFERENCE LIST

Directions: Begin this activity by identifying several people whom you may use as a job or personal reference. Then write the reference information on the lines below. When you have completed your health care reference list to your satisfaction, show it to your instructor for evaluation. Use the sample reference list in Figure 1-1-6 in Section 1, Step 1, as a guide to create your reference list. Then key your final reference list and save the file on the same disk as your resume. Print your final reference list on white 8-1/2 x 11" paper, the same quality used for your resume. Place your printed reference list and computer disk with the resume file in your employment portfolio for easy updating and future reference.

REFERENCES OF (Your Name) _____

_____
Name   Title

_____
Business/Health Care Organization Name

_____
Number and Street Name

_____
City   State   Zip Code

_____
(Area Code) Telephone Number

_____
Name   Title

_____
Business/Health Care Organization Name

_____
Number and Street Name

_____
City   State   Zip Code

_____
(Area Code) Telephone Number

_____

Name   Title

_____

Business/Health Care Organization Name

_____

Number and Street Name

_____

City   State   Zip Code

_____

(Area Code) Telephone Number

_____

Name   Title

_____

Business/Health Care Organization Name

_____

Number and Street Name

_____

City   State   Zip Code

_____

(Area Code) Telephone Number

_____

Name   Title

_____

Business/Health Care Organization Name

_____

Number and Street Name

_____

City   State   Zip Code

_____

(Area Code) Telephone Number

_____

Name   Title

_____

Business/Health Care Organization Name

_____

Number and Street Name

_____

City   State   Zip Code

_____

(Area Code) Telephone Number

Name _____ Date _____

SECTION 1 STEP 2
HEALTH CARE COVER LETTER

ACTIVITY 5
WRITING A HEALTH CARE COVER LETTER

Directions: To complete this activity, first write your practice health care cover letter on this paper. Use the sample cover letters in Figures 1-2-1, 1-2-2, and 1-2-3 in Section 1, Step 2 as guides. Your telephone number, with area code, needs to be shown in your request for an interview, or immediately below your keyed name. Your fax and e-mail address can also be included. When you have drafted your cover letter to your satisfaction, show it to your instructor for evaluation. Next, key your cover letter and save it on the same disk used for your resume. Print your final cover letter on white 8-1/2 x 11" paper, the same quality used for your resume. Place your printed health care cover letter and computer disk in your employment portfolio for future reference.

Your Mailing Address   _____

_____

_____

Date of Letter   _____

Name of Person   _____

Medical Organization Name   _____

Street Address   _____

City, State, Zip Code   _____

Dear _____,

Purpose of Letter   _____

_____

_____

_____

_____

_____

_____

_____

_____

_____

_____

Qualifications or Reasons
Why Applicant Should Be
Interviewed

_____
_____
_____
_____
_____
_____
_____
_____

Request for Interview

_____
_____
_____
_____
_____
_____
_____

Sincerely,

Your Signature

_____

Your Name Keyed

_____

Enclosure

Name _____ Date _____

STEP 3

HEALTH CARE EMPLOYMENT APPLICATION

ACTIVITY 6

COMPLETING A HEALTH CARE EMPLOYMENT APPLICATION

Directions: Use pages 90-93 for the employment applications for Delta Memorial Hospital and Pacific Medical Center. Choose one to complete. When you have neatly completed this activity, show it to your instructor for evaluation. Then place it in your employment portfolio for future reference when completing other employment applications.

DMH

DELTA MEMORIAL HOSPITAL

APPLICATION FOR EMPLOYMENT

TYPE OR PRINT CLEARLY

LAST | FIRST | MIDDLE

PERSONAL INFORMATION

DATE ______ SOCIAL SECURITY NUMBER ______

NAME ______ LAST ______ FIRST ______ MIDDLE

PRESENT ADDRESS ______ STREET ______ CITY ______ STATE ______ ZIP CODE

PERMANENT ADDRESS ______ STREET ______ CITY ______ STATE ______ ZIP CODE

PHONE NO. ______

CAN YOU, AFTER EMPLOYMENT, SUBMIT VERIFICATION OF YOUR LEGAL RIGHT TO WORK IN THE UNITED STATES? CIRCLE ONE: YES NO (IF YES, VERIFICATION WILL BE REQUIRED)

EMPLOYMENT DESIRED

POSITION ______ DATE YOU CAN START ______ SALARY DESIRED ______

ARE YOU EMPLOYED NOW? ______ IF SO MAY WE INQUIRE OF YOUR PRESENT EMPLOYER ______

EDUCATION	NAME AND LOCATION OF SCHOOL	DEGREE OR CERTIFICATE	SUBJECTS STUDIED
HIGH SCHOOL			
UNIVERSITY OR COLLEGE			
TRADE, BUSINESS, OR CORRESPONDENCE SCHOOL			

DO YOU HAVE ANY EXPERIENCES, SKILLS, OR QUALIFICATIONS THAT WILL BE OF SPECIAL BENEFIT IN THE POSITION FOR WHICH YOU ARE APPLYING? ______

WHAT FOREIGN LANGUAGES DO YOU SPEAK FLUENTLY? ______

READ? ______ WRITE? ______

WHAT PROFESSIONAL ORGANIZATIONS DO YOU BELONG TO? ______

CONTINUED ON OTHER SIDE

Figure 3-3-1 Application for employment at Delta Memorial Hospital (Front)

WORK EXPERIENCE

List all present and past employment, including part-time or seasonal, beginning with the most recent.

Employer	Employment Dates and Salary	Describe the work you did in detail	Reason for leaving
Name_____ Address_____ City_____ State_____ Phone_____Supervisor_____	From: _____ To: _____ Salary _____		
Name_____ Address_____ City_____ State_____ Phone_____Supervisor_____	From: _____ To: _____ Salary _____		
Name_____ Address_____ City_____ State_____ Phone_____Supervisor_____	From: _____ To: _____ Salary _____		
Name_____ Address_____ City_____ State_____ Phone_____Supervisor_____	From: _____ To: _____ Salary _____		

REFERENCES: GIVE BELOW THE NAMES OF THREE PERSONS NOT RELATED TO YOU, WHOM YOU HAVE KNOWN AT LEAST ONE YEAR.

NAME	ADDRESS	BUSINESS	YEARS ACQUAINTED
1			
2			
3			

IN CASE OF
EMERGENCY NOTIFY _____
NAME

_____
ADDRESS   PHONE NO.

I AUTHORIZE INVESTIGATION OF ALL STATEMENTS CONTAINED IN THIS APPLICATION. I UNDERSTAND THAT MISREPRESENTATION OR OMISSION OF FACTS CALLED FOR IS CAUSE FOR DISMISSAL. FURTHER, I UNDERSTAND AND AGREE THAT MY EMPLOYMENT IS FOR NO DEFINITE PERIOD AND MAY, REGARDLESS OF THE DATE OF PAYMENT OF MY WAGES AND SALARY, BE TERMINATED AT ANY TIME WITHOUT ANY PREVIOUS NOTICE.

DATE _____ SIGNATURE _____

Figure 3-3-1 Application for employment at Delta Memorial Hospital (Back)

PACIFIC MEDICAL CENTER

EMPLOYMENT APPLICATION

PLEASE TYPE OR PRINT LEGIBLY.
FILL IN ALL AREAS COMPLETELY.

THE PACIFIC MEDICAL CENTER PROGRAM IS AN EQUAL OPPORTUNITY EMPLOYER. FACTS RELATING TO YOUR RACE, COLOR, RELIGION, NATIONAL ORIGIN, SEX, OR AGE ARE NOT CONSIDERED IN DETERMINING YOUR QUALIFICATIONS FOR EMPLOYMENT.

PERSONAL

LAST NAME	FIRST	MIDDLE	TODAY'S DATE

HOW REFERRED TO PACIFIC MEDICAL CENTER?	SOCIAL SECURITY NUMBER	HOME PHONE	WORK/MSG PHONE

CURRENT ADDRESS-STREET | CITY | STATE | ZIP CODE | HOW LONG — YRS. MOS.

PREVIOUS ADDRESS-STREET | CITY | STATE | ZIP CODE | HOW LONG — YRS. MOS.

POSITION APPLIED FOR | SALARY DESIRED | DATE AVAILABLE FOR WORK

ARE YOU WILLING TO WORK:
☐ Days ☐ Evenings ☐ Nights ☐ Weekends ☐ Full Time ☐ On Call

ARE YOU WILLING TO ACCEPT TEMPORARY WORK OF:
☐ 60 Days ☐ 90 Days ☐ No

HAVE YOU EVER BEEN CONVICTED OF A CRIME   YES   NO | IF YES, EXPLAIN WHEN, WHERE, AND DISPOSITION OF CASE

IN CASE OF EMERGENCY PLEASE CALL

LAST NAME	FIRST	HOME PHONE	BUS. PHONE

ADDRESS-STREET | CITY | STATE | ZIP CODE

EDUCATIONAL HISTORY

TYPE OF SCHOOL (HIGH SCHOOL, JR. COLLEGE, COLLEGE OR PROFESSIONAL)	SCHOOL NAME AND ADDRESS	ACADEMIC SUBJECT	NO. YEARS ATTENDED	CIRCLE HIGHEST YEARS OF EDUCATION COMPLETED
				1 2 3 4 5 6 7 8 9 10 11 12
				13 14 15 16 17 18
				DEGREE RECEIVED

LIST ALL TRADE OR VOCATIONAL SCHOOLS ATTENDED	DATE COMPLETED	MAJOR SUBJECT	FOREIGN LANGUAGE	SPEAK	READ	WRITE
				GOOD FAIR POOR	GOOD FAIR POOR	GOOD FAIR POOR
				GOOD FAIR POOR	GOOD FAIR POOR	GOOD FAIR POOR
				GOOD FAIR POOR	GOOD FAIR POOR	GOOD FAIR POOR
				GOOD FAIR POOR	GOOD FAIR POOR	GOOD FAIR POOR
			AMESLAN (Am. Sign Language)	GOOD FAIR POOR		

SCHOLASTIC HONORS RECEIVED

PROFESSIONAL

DO YOU HAVE OR HAVE YOU EVER APPLIED FOR A PROFESSIONAL LICENSE, CERTIFICATE, OR REGISTRATION?   ☐ YES   ☐ NO

NUMBER	TYPE	DATE OF EXPIRATION	IF PENDING, GIVE DATE APPLICATION STARTED

IN WHAT PROFESSIONAL ASSOCIATIONS DO YOU MAINTAIN MEMBERSHIP?

CONTINUED ON OTHER SIDE

Figure 3-3-2 Application for employment at Pacific Medical Center (Front)

EMPLOYED	LIST LAST EMPLOYER FIRST	JOB DESCRIPTION AND TITLE	RATE OF PAY	REASON FOR LEAVING
FROM Month Year	NAME OF EMPLOYER	TITLE	START	
	STREET ADDRESS	DUTIES		
	CITY, STATE, ZIP			
TO Month Year	TELEPHONE NUMBER		LAST	
	NAME OF SUPERVISOR			
FROM Month Year	NAME OF EMPLOYER	TITLE	START	
	STREET ADDRESS	DUTIES		
	CITY, STATE, ZIP			
TO Month Year	TELEPHONE NUMBER		LAST	
	NAME OF SUPERVISOR			
FROM Month Year	NAME OF EMPLOYER	TITLE	START	
	STREET ADDRESS	DUTIES		
	CITY, STATE, ZIP			
TO Month Year	TELEPHONE NUMBER		LAST	
	NAME OF SUPERVISOR			
FROM Month Year	NAME OF EMPLOYER	TITLE	START	
	STREET ADDRESS	DUTIES		
	CITY, STATE, ZIP			
TO Month Year	TELEPHONE NUMBER		LAST	
	NAME OF SUPERVISOR			

Have you ever worked for any subsidiary of the Pacific Medical Center? ☐ YES ☐ NO   If yes, last date of employment?   Where?   If presently employed may we contact your employer? ☐ YES ☐ NO

Have you ever worked under another name? ☐ YES ☐ NO   If yes, what name(s)   Which co. or organization

SPEEDWRITING SPEED ___ WPM   SHORTHAND SPEED ___ WPM   NET KEYBOARDING SPEED ___ WPM   OTHER MACHINES OPERATED SKILLFULLY

M E D I C A L S T A T U S

This employer is a government contractor subject to section 503 of the Rehabilitation Act of 1973, which requires government contractors to take affirmative action to employ and advance in employment qualified handicapped individuals. If you have such a handicap, and would like to be considered under the affirmative action program, please tell us. This information is voluntary and refusal to provide it will not subject you to rejection for employment, discharge or other disciplinary treatment. However, in order to assure proper placement of all employees, we do request that you answer the following questions:

Do you have or have you had a mental or physical disability which would create a hazard to you or to others at the worksite?   ☐ Yes   ☐ No

If yes, please describe _____

R E F E R E N C E S

NAME 3 PERSONS NOT RELATED TO YOU WHO CAN ATTEST TO YOUR EXPERIENCE AND QUALIFICATIONS

NAME	ADDRESS	CITY	STATE	ZIP CODE	PHONE NO.	OCCUPATION

THE ABOVE INFORMATION IS TRUE AND CORRECT TO THE BEST OF MY KNOWLEDGE. MISREPRESENTATION OR OMISSION OF MATERIAL FACTS (I.E., FACTS RELATED TO MY QUALIFICATIONS FOR THE POSITION FOR WHICH I AM APPLYING) IS CAUSE FOR SEPARATION FROM THE EMPLOYER. I FURTHER AUTHORIZE ALL FORMER EMPLOYERS, SCHOOLS (PROFESSIONAL AND VOCATIONAL), AND PERSONS NAMED ABOVE TO FURNISH REFERENCES AND ANY FACTS WHICH MAY BE PERTINENT TO MY EMPLOYMENT. I UNDERSTAND THAT EMPLOYMENT IS ALSO CONTINGENT UPON PASSING A PHYSICAL EXAMINATION.

Employment with the Pacific Medical Center is voluntarily entered into and the employee is free to resign at any time. Similarly, the Pacific Medical Center may, at any time, conclude the employment relationship where it believes it is in the company's best interest.

_____   _____
(SIGNATURE)   (DATE SIGNED)

Figure 3-3-2 Application for employment at Pacific Medical Center (Back)

Name _____ Date _____

SECTION 1 STEP 4
FINDING AND RESEARCHING
A HEALTH CARE JOB AND FACILITY

ACTIVITY 7
FINDING HEALTH CARE JOB LEADS

Directions: To find health care job leads, record your employment contacts, phone and fax numbers, addresses, and important remarks on the forms provided here. When you have completed your health care job lead information, show it to your instructor for evaluation. Place these contacts in your employment portfolio to help with future leads.

Job Lead 1: School Placement Office

Name of Health Care Facility _____
Contact Person _____
Phone _____ Fax _____ E-mail Address _____
Address _____
City _____ State _____ Zip _____
Remarks _____
_____

Name of Health Care Facility _____
Contact Person _____
Phone _____ Fax _____ E-mail Address _____
Address _____
City _____ State _____ Zip _____
Remarks _____
_____

Job Lead 2: Market Survey

Name of Health Care Facility _____
Contact Person _____
Phone _____ Fax _____ E-mail Address _____
Address _____
City _____ State _____ Zip _____
Remarks _____
_____

Name of Health Care Facility _____
Contact Person _____
Phone _____ Fax _____ E-mail Address _____
Address _____
City _____ State _____ Zip _____
Remarks _____
_____

Job Lead 3: Associations

Name of Health Care Facility _____

Contact Person _____

Phone _____ Fax _____ E-mail Address _____

Address _____

City _____ State _____ Zip _____

Remarks _____

_____

Name of Health Care Facility _____

Contact Person _____

Phone _____ Fax _____ E-mail Address _____

Address _____

City _____ State _____ Zip _____

Remarks _____

_____

Job Lead 4: Networking

Name of Health Care Facility _____

Contact Person _____

Phone _____ Fax _____ E-mail Address _____

Address _____

City _____ State _____ Zip _____

Remarks _____

_____

Name of Health Care Facility _____

Contact Person _____

Phone _____ Fax _____ E-mail Address _____

Address _____

City _____ State _____ Zip _____

Remarks _____

_____

Job Lead 5: Newspaper Employment Ads

Name of Health Care Facility _____

Contact Person _____

Phone _____ Fax _____ E-mail Address _____

Address _____

City _____ State _____ Zip _____

Remarks _____

_____

Name of Health Care Facility _____

Contact Person _____

Phone _____ Fax _____ E-mail Address _____

Address _____

City _____ State _____ Zip _____

Remarks _____

_____

Job Lead 6: Private Employment Agencies

Name of Health Care Facility _____

Contact Person _____

Phone _____ Fax _____ E-mail Address _____

Address _____

City _____ State _____ Zip _____

Remarks _____

_____

Name of Health Care Facility _____

Contact Person _____

Phone _____ Fax _____ E-mail Address _____

Address _____

City _____ State _____ Zip _____

Remarks _____

_____

Job Lead 7: Temporary Employment Agencies

Name of Health Care Facility _____

Contact Person _____

Phone _____ Fax _____ E-mail Address _____

Address _____

City _____ State _____ Zip _____

Remarks _____

_____

Name of Health Care Facility _____

Contact Person _____

Phone _____ Fax _____ E-mail Address _____

Address _____

City _____ State _____ Zip _____

Remarks _____

_____

Job Lead 8: State Employment Office

Name of Health Care Facility _____

Contact Person _____

Phone _____ Fax _____ E-mail Address _____

Address _____

City _____ State _____ Zip _____

Remarks _____

_____

Name of Health Care Facility _____

Contact Person _____

Phone _____ Fax _____ E-mail Address _____

Address _____

City _____ State _____ Zip _____

Remarks _____

_____

Job Lead 9: U.S. Civil Service Employment Office

Name of Health Care Facility _____

Contact Person _____

Phone _____ Fax _____ E-mail Address _____

Address _____

City _____ State _____ Zip _____

Remarks _____

_____

Name of Health Care Facility _____

Contact Person _____

Phone _____ Fax _____ E-mail Address _____

Address _____

City _____ State _____ Zip _____

Remarks _____

_____

Job Lead 10: Your Internet Job Search

Name of Health Care Facility _____

Contact Person _____

Phone _____ Fax _____ E-mail Address _____

Address _____

City _____ State _____ Zip _____

Remarks _____

_____

Name of Health Care Facility _____

Contact Person _____

Phone _____ Fax _____ E-mail Address _____

Address _____

City _____ State _____ Zip _____

Remarks _____

_____

Name _____ Date _____

SECTION 1 STEP 4
FINDING AND RESEARCHING A HEALTH CARE JOB AND FACILITY

ACTIVITY 8
RESEARCHING A HEALTH CARE FACILITY

Directions: To complete this activity, first select one to three health care facilities you would like to research. Be aware that some health care facilities, especially smaller ones, may not have much information written about them. If that is the case, you could write, telephone, or E-mail the health care facility with your questions. If convenient, you could also visit the facility.

Answer the questions that are provided in this activity for each health care facility you select. Do your research at your school library, career center, or your local library. To find publicly owned health care facility information, remember to use the publications and magazines suggested in Section 1, Step 4. If possible, use the Internet as well. When you have completed the research to your satisfaction, show it to your instructor for evaluation. Place your completed research in your employment portfolio. In the future, this activity will help you research medical organizations for important information and know what questions you need to answer before any job interview.

Health Care Facility Name _____

What services does this health care facility provide? _____
_____
_____

What kinds of health care jobs do they have? _____
_____
_____

How old is this health care facility? _____

In what cities does this medical organization have facilities? _____
_____
_____

What is the size of this health care facility? Is it growing or shrinking in number of employees?
_____

Who are this health care facility's competitors? _____
_____
_____

Questions I have about this health care organization: _____

_____

_____

Health Care Facility Name _____

What services does this health care facility provide? _____

_____

_____

What kinds of health care jobs do they have? _____

_____

_____

How old is this health care facility? _____

In what cities does this medical organization have facilities? _____

_____

_____

What is the size of this health care facility? Is it growing or shrinking in number of employees?

_____

Who are this health care facility's competitors? _____

_____

_____

Questions I have about this health care organization: _____

_____

_____

Health Care Facility Name _____

What services does this health care facility provide? _____

_____

_____

What kinds of health care jobs do they have? _____

_____

_____

How old is this health care facility? _____

In what cities does this medical organization have facilities? _____

_____

_____

What is the size of this health care facility? Is it growing or shrinking in number of employees?

_____

Who are this health care facility's competitors? _____

_____

_____

Questions I have about this health care organization: _____

_____

_____

Name _____ Date _____

SECTION 1 STEP 5
HOW TO PREPARE FOR A HEALTH CARE INTERVIEW

ACTIVITY 9
ANSWERING INTERVIEW QUESTIONS

Directions: To complete this activity, remember to have a particular job and health care facility in mind. Then, using your own words, write answers to each interview question. You may also use the suggested answers in Section 1, Step 5 to help you answer the health care interview questions. When you have completed the answers, show them to your instructor for evaluation. Then work in groups to practice answering the questions with your written replies.

1. In what type of health care position are you most interested?

_____
_____
_____
_____

2. Why do you want to leave your current job? *or* Why did you leave your last job?

_____
_____
_____
_____

3. What pay do you expect?

_____
_____
_____
_____

4. Why do you want to work for our health care facility?

_____
_____
_____
_____

5. Have you had any serious illness or injury that might prevent you from performing your duties in this health care position?

_____
_____
_____
_____

6. Do you have references?

_____

_____

_____

_____

7. What did you like _best_ or _least_ about your last job?

_____

_____

_____

_____

8. Are you looking for a permanent or temporary job? Do you want full-time or part-time employment?

_____

_____

_____

_____

9. Tell me something about yourself. Why do you think we should hire you for this health care position?

_____

_____

_____

_____

10. How well do you work under pressure?

_____

_____

_____

_____

11. What are your strengths and weaknesses?

_____

_____

_____

_____

12. What are your short-term and long-term employment goals?

_____

_____

_____

_____

Name _____ Date _____

SECTION 1 STEP 6
DURING THE HEALTH CARE INTERVIEW

CTIVITY 10
HEALTH CARE CASE STUDY QUESTIONS

Directions: Carefully review the model health care interview between Maria Lopez and Mr. Robert Allen in Section 1, Step 6. Since this is a model interview you should become very familiar with the answers and practice them before your next interview. When you have completed the case study answers to your satisfaction, show them to your instructor for evaluation. Now answer the following questions.

1. Make a list of six facts that Maria knows about the health care position after the interview.

   a. _____
   b. _____
   c. _____
   d. _____
   e. _____
   f. _____

2. Make a list of six facts that Mr. Robert Allen knows about Maria after the interview.

   a. _____
   b. _____
   c. _____
   d. _____
   e. _____
   f. _____

3. How did Maria attempt to convince Mr. Allen that her lack of medical transcription employment was not important in considering her for the job opening?

   _____

   _____

4. In the interview, how did Maria say that her school classes helped her?

   _____

   _____

For a future interview, tell how your school classes have helped you.

_____

_____

5. What was Maria's answer to Mr. Allen's question, "Why would you want to work for Danville Health Center?"

_____

_____

How would you have answered this question if you were Maria?

_____

_____

6. What was Maria's answer when Mr. Allen asked if she enjoyed working for Hammond's Discount Bookstore?

_____

_____

7. What answer did Maria give to Mr. Allen's question, "What pay do you expect?"

_____

_____

8. How does Maria plan to follow up her interview with Mr. Allen?

_____

_____

What follow-up technique would you have used? Why?

_____

_____

9. Reread the end of Maria's conversation with Mr. Allen. Was it too short? Was it complimentary? What would you add or take out?

_____

_____

10. If Mr. Allen should decide to hire Maria, would you feel he had matched the right person to this health care position? Why or why not?

_____

_____

Name _____ Date _____

SECTION 1 STEP 7
AFTER THE HEALTH CARE INTERVIEW

ACTIVITY 11
PREPARING A HEALTH CARE POST-INTERVIEW LETTER

Directions: To complete this activity, first write your practice post-interview letter below using the sample post-interview letter in Figure 1-7-1, in Section 1, Step 7 as a guide. When you have drafted your letter to your satisfaction, show it to your instructor for evaluation. Next, using this completed draft, key your post-interview letter following the spacing guidelines given in the sample post-interview letter. Place your keyed post-interview letter along with the computer disk in your employment portfolio for future reference.

Your Mailing Address _____

_____

Date of Letter _____

Name of Person _____

Title of Person _____

Company Name _____

Street Address _____

City, State, Zip Code _____

Dear _____,

Thank You and _____
Positive Comment
about Interview _____

_____

_____

_____

_____

_____

_____

Emphasize Strengths   _____

_____

_____

_____

_____

_____

_____

_____

_____

Continued Interest
and Additional
Reasons for Hiring   _____

_____

_____

_____

_____

_____

_____

_____

Sincerely,

Your Signature   _____

Your Name Keyed
Your Area Code
and Phone Number   _____

_____

_____

Name _____ Date _____

SECTION 2 STEP 1
QUESTIONS TO CONSIDER BEFORE LEAVING A HEALTH CARE JOB

CTIVITY 12
HEALTH CARE CASE STUDY—DECISION TIME

Directions: Read the following case study on Peter Chang who wants to make a decision about leaving his health care job. In the space provided write the advantages and disadvantages of Peter staying in his current health care position and answer the questions that follow. When you have completed the answers to your satisfaction, show it to your instructor for evaluation and class discussion. Then place this activity in your employment portfolio for future reference.

Peter Chang has been employed by Maumee Medical Center, a large health maintenance organization, as a medical assistant for almost three years. At first he was happy with his health care job. He enjoyed his independence and the environment of the health care facility. Now, Peter goes home most nights with a splitting headache. His doctor recently told him that his blood pressure was up and he should relax more. Peter's problems developed when the Maumee Medical Center started making changes in the last year. Peter has a new supervisor, who often questions how he does things. Worse, one person, who started working there after Peter, was promoted. Peter felt he was ready for the assistant supervisor position the person received. Also, the health care facility is much more rigid than when he started. There are more paperwork duties and rules to follow than before. While he is not happy with the work environment, Peter still enjoys his work. He is also thinking about becoming trained as an X-ray technician on new, state-of-the-art equipment that has just been installed. Peter thinks he should just quit, but then he remembers that his car loan will not be paid off for another year. In two years he will be fully eligible for the health care facility's profit sharing and savings plan.

1. From the case study, identify at least three advantages and three disadvantages to Peter's staying in his current health care employment.

Advantages of Staying	Disadvantages of Staying
1. _____	1. _____
_____	_____
2. _____	2. _____
_____	_____
3. _____	3. _____
_____	_____

Other Advantages	Other Disadvantages
_____	_____
_____	_____
_____	_____
_____	_____
_____	_____
_____	_____

2. Do you think Peter should or should not leave his current health care position? Why?

_____

_____

_____

_____

_____

_____

_____

_____

_____

_____

_____

_____

3. If you decide he should stay, list three things Peter could do to improve his health care job situation.

_____

_____

_____

_____

_____

_____

_____

_____

_____

_____

_____

_____

_____

_____

_____

_____

Name _____ Date _____

SECTION 2 STEP 2

THE BEST WAY TO LEAVE A HEALTH CARE JOB

CTIVITY 13

WRITING A HEALTH CARE RESIGNATION LETTER

Directions: To complete this activity, first write your practice health care resignation letter below. Use the sample health care resignation letter in Figure 2-2-2, in Section 2, Step 2 of this manual as a guide. When you have drafted the letter to your satisfaction, show it to your instructor for evaluation. Next, using this completed draft, key your resignation letter. Save the health care resignation letter file on your resume disk. Print your final health care resignation letter on the same quality paper used for your resume. Place your printed resignation letter and computer disk in your employment portfolio for future reference.

Your Mailing Address   _____

_____

_____

Date of Letter   _____

Name of Person   _____
Title of Person   _____
Health Care Facility Name   _____
Street Address   _____
City, State, Zip Code   _____

Dear _____,

Date of Resignation   _____

_____

Reason(s) for Leaving   _____

_____

Appreciation of
Skills Learned   _____

Appreciation of Fellow
Employees or Health
Care Facility   _____

_____

Sincerely,

Your Signature   _____

Your Name Keyed   _____

Name _____ Date _____

SECTION 2 STEP 2
THE BEST WAY TO LEAVE A HEALTH CARE JOB

ACTIVITY 14
HEALTH CARE EXIT CONVERSATION

Directions: Complete this activity by writing your practice health care exit conversation below. Use the sample health care exit conversation in Section 2, Step 2 as a guide. Notice the positive remarks in this example and construct your own positive health care exit conversation. Try to make this as relevant as possible to your situation by having in mind your present or a past employer. When you have completed the written conversation to your satisfaction, show it to your instructor for evaluation. Place your written health care exit conversation in your employment portfolio for future reference.

Notice of Resignation and Reason(s) for Leaving

_____
_____
_____

Positive Comments about Health Care Work Experience (Health Care Facility or Co-workers)

_____
_____
_____

Statement of Health Care Job Skills Learned/Work Habits Improved

_____
_____
_____

Offer to Train Replacement

_____
_____
_____

Name _____ Date _____

SECTION 2 STEP **3**
HEALTH CARE REFERENCE LETTER

CTIVITY 15
CONSTRUCTING A HEALTH CARE REFERENCE LETTER

Directions: To complete this activity, first write your practice reference letter below. Use the sample reference letter in Figure 2-3-1 in Section 2, Step 3 as a guide. You may want to use the name of your present or a past employer as your reference. When you have drafted the letter to your satisfaction, show it to your instructor for evaluation. Next, using this completed draft, key your reference letter and save the file to the same disk on which you have your resume and other job-related documents. Print your final reference letter on the same quality paper used for your resume. Have your reference person sign the letter and then place the keyed reference letter and computer disk in your employment portfolio for future reference.

Reference letters from employers should be on company letterhead

LINCOLN
MEDICAL CENTER
482 Concord Drive / Lincoln, NE 68502-4901
(402) 555-2888

Date of Letter   _____

                                  Dear Hiring Manager,

Abilities, Skills, and   _____
Accomplishments   _____
                                  _____
                                  _____
                                  _____

Attitudes   _____
and Character   _____
                                  _____

Invitation to Reader   _____
to Call for More   _____
Details
                                  Sincerely,

Signature of Employer   _____

(Keyed)
Name of Employer   _____
Title of Employer   _____

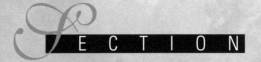

4

Using the
CD-ROM

INTRODUCTION

Your CD-ROM contains 18 files that you may use to supplement *How to Get a Job in Health Care* activities and complete your resume and letter documents. The chart shown here gives the title and CD-ROM file name, section and step number, and specific directions for each of the CD-ROM files listed. Always save the file to your computer disk and place a copy in your employment portfolio for future employment assistance.

Your CD-ROM also includes the Health Care Resume Generator. After entering your personal information, this easy-to-use software will generate a variety of personalized resumes and cover letters designed specifically to help you find a rewarding job in the health care field.

Section 1 Step	Title *File Name*	Directions
1	Standard Resume *Standard Resume.doc* Chronological Resume *Chronological Resume.doc* Functional Resume *Functional Resume.doc* Combination Resume *Combination Resume.doc*	Four health care resume formats appear on your computer screen. Select and edit the health care resume that is appropriate for you. Use your corresponding resume activity practice sheet for editing information. DO NOT EDIT RESUME HEADINGS. Supply your personal information under each heading. Maintain suggested resume spacing when editing your resume.
1	Reference List *Reference List.doc*	A reference list format appears on your computer screen. Edit this reference list, keeping the main heading and using the suggested spacing.
2	Cover Letter Planner *Cover Letter Planner.doc*	Before keying your health care cover letter, use this planner to outline your main cover letter points. Keep in mind that the primary objective of a cover letter is to secure an interview.
2	Cover Letter 1 *Cover Letter 1.doc* Cover Letter 2 *Cover Letter 2.doc* Cover Letter 3.doc *Cover letter 3.doc*	Three health care cover letter formats appear on your computer screen. Select and edit the health care cover letter that is appropriate for you. Use information from your CD-ROM cover letter planner and corresponding Section 3 cover letter activity practice sheet for editing. Maintain suggested spacing when editing your cover letter.
4	Job Search Planner *Job Search Planner.doc*	A successful health care job search requires organization and effort. The weekly planner allows you to set goals for generating a number of health care job leads, setting up a specific number of interviews, or making contact with a specific health care facility.
5, 6, 7	Interview Planner *Interview Planner.doc*	During an extensive job search you may find it difficult to remember details of every meeting. That is why it is important to develop a record keeping system for all your interviews. This planner records details, reminders, notes, and contacts.
7	Post Interview Letter Planner *Post Interview Letter Planner.doc*	Before writing your post-interview letter, you may find it helpful to determine your key points. This planner helps you identify what is important to say in your post-interview letter.

(continues)

Section 1 Step	Title *File Name*	Directions
7	Post Interview Letter *Post Interview Letter.doc*	A sample post-interview letter appears on your computer screen. Edit this letter using information from your CD-ROM post-interview letter planner and your Section 3 practice activity sheet. Maintain suggested spacing when editing your post-interview letter.
7	Job Offer Evaluator *Job Offer Evaluator.doc*	Te decision to accept or reject a health care job offer is an important one. This job offer evaluator helps you make a decision about one job or helps you compare several offers.

Section 2 Step	Title *File Name*	Directions
2	Exit Conversation and Resignation Letter Planner *Exit Conversation and Resignation Letter Planner.doc*	Before writing a resignation letter or having an exit conversation with your employer, good planning will ensure your leaving is positive. This planner helps you organize your thoughts.
2	Resignation Letter *Resignation Letter.doc*	A sample resignation letter appears on your computer screen. Edit this letter using information from your CD-ROM resignation letter planner and your Section 3 resignation letter practice activity sheet. Maintain suggested spacing when editing your resignation letter.
3	Reference Letter Planner *Reference Letter Planner.doc*	When you are given permission to draft a letter of reference about yourself for someone else's signature, put yourself in that person's shoes. This planner will help you outline how someone sees you.
3	Reference Letter *Reference Letter.doc*	A sample health care reference letter appears on your computer screen. Edit this letter using information from your CD-ROM reference letter planner and your Section 3 reference letter practice activity.

Using Delmar's Health Care Resume Generator CD-ROM

To use the Health Care Resume Generator program on the CD-ROM, you need to have Microsoft® Word 97 or later installed on your computer.

System Requirements

Microsoft® Word 97 or later
Operating system: Microsoft® Windows® 95 or better
Processor: Pentium or faster
Memory: 24 MB or more
Hard disk space: 24 MB or more
CD-ROM drive: 2x

Setup Instructions

1. Insert the disk into your CD-ROM player
2. From the Start Menu, choose **Run**
3. In the **Open** text box, enter **d:\ setup.exe** then click the **OK** button (Substitute the letter of your CD-ROM drive for **d:**)
4. Follow the installation prompts from there

Technical Support

For technical support with Delmar's Health Care Resume Generator CD-ROM, please call 800-477-3692 or email Delmar Learning at help@delmar.com.

License Agreement for Delmar Learning, a division of Thomson Learning, Inc.

Educational Software/Data

You the customer, and Delmar Learning, a division of Thomson Learning, Inc. incur certain benefits, rights, and obligations to each other when you open this package and use the software/data it contains. BE SURE YOU READ THE LICENSE AGREEMENT CAREFULLY, SINCE BY USING THE SOFTWARE/DATA YOU INDICATE YOU HAVE READ, UNDERSTOOD, AND ACCEPTED THE TERMS OF THIS AGREEMENT.

Your rights:

1. You enjoy a non-exclusive license to use the software/data on a single microcomputer in consideration for payment of the required license fee, (which may be included in the purchase price of an accompanying print component), or receipt of this software/data, and your acceptance of the terms and conditions of this agreement.

2. You acknowledge that you do not own the aforesaid software/data. You also acknowledge that the software/data is furnished "as is," and contains copyrighted and/or proprietary and confidential information of Delmar Learning, a division of Thomson Learning, Inc. or its licensors.

There are limitations on your rights:

1. You may not copy or print the software/data for any reason whatsoever, except to install it on a hard drive on a single microcomputer and to make one archival copy, unless copying or printing is expressly permitted in writing or statements recorded on the diskette(s).

2. You may not revise, translate, convert, disassemble or otherwise reverse engineer the software/data except that you may add to or rearrange any data recorded on the media as part of the normal use of the software/data.

3. You may not sell, license, lease, rent, loan or otherwise distribute or network the software/data except that you may give the software/data to a student or and instructor for use at school or, temporarily at home.

Should you fail to abide by the Copyright Law of the United States as it applies to this software/data your license to use it will become invalid. You agree to erase or otherwise destroy the software/data immediately after receiving note of termination of this agreement for violation of its provisions from Delmar Learning.

Delmar Learning, a division of Thomson Learning, Inc gives you a LIMITED WARRANTY covering the enclosed software/data. The LIMITED WARRANTY follows this License.

This license is the entire agreement between you and Delmar Learning, a division of Thomson Learning, Inc. interpreted and enforced under New York law.

LIMITED WARRANTY

Delmar Learning, a division of Thomson Learning, Inc. warrants to the original licensee/purchaser of this copy of microcomputer software/data and the media on which it is recorded that the media will be free from defects in material and workmanship for ninety (90) days from the date of original purchase. All implied warranties are limited in duration to this ninety (90) day period. THEREAFTER, ANY IMPLIED WARRANTIES, INCLUDING IMPLIED WARRANTIES OF MERCHANTABILITY AND FITNESS FOR A PARTICULAR PURPOSE, ARE EXCLUDED. THIS WARRANTY IS IN LIEU OF ALL OTHER WARRANTIES, WHETHER ORAL OR WRITTEN, EXPRESS OR IMPLIED.

If you believe the media is defective please return it during the ninety day period to the address shown below. Defective media will be replaced without charge provided that it has not been subjected to misuse or damage.

This warranty does not extend to the software or information recorded on the media. The software and information are provided "AS IS." Any statements made about the utility of the software or information are not to be considered as express or implied warranties.

Limitation of liability: Our liability to you for any losses shall be limited to direct damages, and shall not exceed the amount you paid for the software. In no event will we be liable to you for any indirect, special, incidental, or consequential damages (including loss of profits) even if we have been advised of the possibility of such damages.

Some states do not allow the exclusion or limitation of incidental or consequential damages, or limitations on the duration of implied warranties, so the above limitation or exclusion may not apply to you. This warranty gives you specific legal rights, and you may also have other rights which vary from state to state. Address all correspondence to: Delmar Learning, a division of Thomson Learning, Inc., 5 Maxwell Drive, P.O. Box 8007, Clifton Park, NY 12065-8007. Attention: Technology Department